The Psychotherapy
Documentation Primer
Second Edition

The Psychotherapy
Documentation Primer
Second Edition

DONALD E. WIGER

WILEY

JOHN WILEY & SONS, INC.

Note about Photocopy Rights

The publisher grants purchasers permission to reproduce handouts from this book for professional
use with their clients.

Library of Congress Cataloging-in-Publication Data:

Wiger, Donald E., 1953–
    The psychotherapy documentation primer / Donald E. Wiger. — 2nd ed.
        p. cm. — (Practice planners series)
    Includes bibliographical references and index.
    ISBN-13 978-0-471-73016-3 (pbk.)
    ISBN-10 0-471-73016-5 (pbk.)
    1. Psychiatric records. 2. Mental health services—Medical records. 3. Mental health services—
Management. I. Title. II. Practice planners.
    RC455.2.M38W543 2005
    362.2′068—dc22

                                                                        2005043594

Printed in the United States of America

10 9 8 7 6 5 4 3 2 1

This book is dedicated to Helen Lockery of Maplewood, MN.

Mom, I want to thank you for being there consistently all of my life. You have been a blessing to so many people. Perhaps no one has ever thanked you for the sacrifice you chose to make by leaving high school early to help support your family. Now, I will always be there for you. I don't exactly know what it is about you (there are many great things), but you did a great job in raising a son who is a state senator, a daughter who is a hard-working, giving, and warm person, and me. We have all done very well in life because of your example. You taught each of us to make a difference in other people's lives.

Preface

A number of years have passed since writing the first edition of *The Psychotherapy Documentation Primer*. I have presented this material to literally thousands of mental health professionals, who have received the material rather with expressions ranging from, "Thank you, I needed this," to "I entered the field to help people, not fill out paperwork." Typically, those newer to the field welcome the material as part of their clinical training. However, oftentimes seasoned professionals may have difficulty agreeing with a medical model of documentation. Overall, those who review case documentation such as case managers, accreditation agencies, and licensure officials have highly supported the principles taught in the primer.

Although the basic tenets of documentation have not changed significantly since the first edition, the second edition provides a *tune up,* enabling the reader to run on the course of documentation more easily. This edition provides more examples and explanations of documentation materials, plus it adds a Health Insurance Portability and Accountability Act (HIPAA) component.

This author enjoys presenting this material to agencies across the country in seminar form and can be reached through the Minnesota School of Professional Psychology or through the publisher, John Wiley & Sons, for groups interested in documentation training.

DONALD E. WIGER

Contents

1

Introduction

We are living in the age of professional accountability. In addition to mental health workers, professionals such as politicians, executives, clergy, educators, and people from most walks of life have increasing demands placed on them to demonstrate that they have practiced their profession effectively and ethically. In the past few years an increasing number of well-known public figures have filled the headlines and court dockets due to compromising their professional standards. Colleges and professional schools have increased the number of their required ethics courses. Many mental health licensing boards require ongoing ethical training as part of their mandatory continuing education.

Standards of accountability in the mental health profession come from a number of sources. State boards, such as psychology, nursing, social work, professional counselors, and marriage and family therapy, each have specific guidelines for licensees. Accrediting agencies, such as the Commission of Accreditation for Rehabilitation Facilities (CARF) and the Joint Commission of Accreditation of Healthcare Organizations (JCAHO), and third-party payers, such as insurance companies and managed care organizations, maintain specific documentation requirements to assure accountability.

Such regulations help curtail the rising costs of mental health services, which have skyrocketed due to factors such as inflation and increased mental health benefits. Current standards of third-party payers hold that services must be medically necessary in order to be covered for payment. Both third-party payers and regulatory agencies impose strict requirements in which each step of the clinical process must be clearly documented. Therefore, appropriate documentation and communicating evidence of clients' needs for services is crucial for a clinic's financial and professional survival.

Learning appropriate documentation procedures goes far beyond meeting professional regulations or requirements for payment of services. Accurate recording procedures provide clear evidence of what takes place in mental health sessions. Without clear documentation, there is not an appropriate record of what takes place in therapy; thus it is difficult to evaluate therapeutic effectiveness. Sloppy clinical procedures are not only unfair to the client but also may border on malpractice. During times such as a third-party audit or a clinical review, proper documentation validates that appropriate treatment took place. When sound documentation procedures are followed, a written record of treatment will be available for review of (a) therapeutic effectiveness, (b) appropriateness of services, (c) continuity of services, and (d) evaluation of therapeutic outcomes, setting a high standard for mental health treatment.

When poor documentation takes place, there is not clear written evidence of the course of therapy. With or without documentation requirements, responsible clinicians will continue to provide clients with valuable services, whereas those who are prone to cutting corners must provide evidence of the effectiveness of their services.

Documentation procedures can directly affect the financial condition of a clinic. It is not uncommon for an insurance provider to audit records. When records do not adequately demonstrate that services were necessary, on target, or concordant with the presenting problem or diagnosis, it is possible that the clinic will have to pay back money received from the insurance company. Such audits have put some clinics out of business.

In the past, third-party payers simply paid therapists when an insurance claim was made. Costs skyrocketed; thus managed care was necessary and subsequently flourished. Today, third-party payers no longer blindly accept billing for any psychotherapy services. They require specific types of evidence demonstrating the client's need for services and the therapeutic effectiveness in order to pay for the treatment. Without knowing proper documentation procedures and how to present a case on paper, the therapist is vulnerable to appearing to be "out of compliance" or providing "unnecessary services" even if the treatment is exceptional.

Although most mental health professionals are properly schooled in conducting psychotherapy, few receive any training in documenting the evidence of their treatment. It is not uncommon for therapists new to the field to become discouraged when exposed to the "other responsibility" of treatment, documentation. However, when properly trained, therapists soon realize the benefits of documentation by not only becoming more confident in meeting third-party requirements but also by becoming more aware of their client's progresses. Learning documentation procedures is a win-win situation.

Documentation is atheoretical. That is, it does not follow a certain theoretical school of thought. It is presented as *behavioral evidence* in measurable terms; however, this has nothing to do with behavioral therapy. The clinician may conduct psychotherapy from any effective type of treatment (e.g., cognitive, behavioral, dynamic, rational-emotive, solutions focused, etc.). Managed care companies, along with other third-party payers and accrediting organizations, are open to this variation, provided that the improvements in client functioning are documented in behavioral terms. The evidence is presented in terms of objective client behaviors, not opinions or speculation. Evidence of alleviation of specific client impairments is required. They question, "What changes in behavior are taking place as the result of therapy?"

Regulatory agencies require that the same measuring stick is used to assess the effects of therapy regardless of the treatment modality employed. The current measurement standards in mental health require that clinical documentation be observable, measurable, and provide behavioral evidence of therapeutic progress.

Documentation begins at the first interview. The several documentation procedures conducted throughout therapy are interrelated. The information collected in the initial interview is necessary for writing the treatment plan. The treatment plan provides a guideline for the course of therapy, which is documented in the progress notes. Progress notes are necessary for writing a revised treatment plan. All of the information collected is needed in writing the discharge summary and assessing outcomes as outlined in Figure 1.1.

The documentation procedure examples provided in this text represent a course of treatment for a client with depression. In addition, Appendix A provides documentation examples for a client with Panic Disorder with Agoraphobia.

This text begins with teaching the rationale and examples of documentation for each step of the therapeutic process. In addition, it provides training as to what documentation is required for third-party payers and accreditation agencies.

FIGURE 1.1
The Course of Documentation

Initial	Diagnostic Interview
	Treatment Plan
	Progress Notes
Cycles of	Treatment Plan Revisions/Updates
	Progress Notes
End	Discharge Summary

HIGHLIGHTS
of Chapter 1

★ Accurate and specific documentation procedures are necessary for ethical, professional, and financial reasons.

★ Third-party payers and accrediting agencies are becoming more stringent in documentation procedures.

★ The intake, treatment plan, progress notes, revised treatment plan, and discharge summary are interrelated. Although they are independent documents, they represent a continuous process in therapy and documentation.

★ Each step in the counseling procedures has specific documentation procedures, which, if not followed, could be detrimental to the client, therapist, and the clinic. Likewise, all can benefit with appropriate procedures.

QUESTIONS

1. In the medical model of documentation, the means by which a therapist documents therapy
    (a) depends on the theoretical school of thought.
    (b) is atheoretical.
    (c) is not important.
    (d) incorporates documenting impairments rather than strengths.

2. A current requirement by most third-party payers to cover mental health services is documenting

    (a) that personal growth will take place in therapy.

    (b) that a preexisting condition was not present.

    (c) proof of insurability.

    (d) medical necessity.

3. Client files that are audited by a third-party payer that are not found to be compliant with documentation standards

    (a) typically leads to loss of licensure.

    (b) is a minor concern to most clinicians.

    (c) may be subject to repaying funds back to the third-party payer.

    (d) is a clear violation of confidentiality.

4. Typically, the evidence a third-party case manager uses to determine that the treatment plan has been followed is found

    (a) in the progress notes.

    (b) by interviewing the client.

    (c) through determining the number of sessions that have been conducted to date.

    (d) in the initial summary report.

Answers: 1. b; 2. d; 3. c; 4. a

2

Overview of Current Documentation Procedures and Third-Party Requirements

Documentation procedures have changed dramatically since the 1980s. Previously, they consisted of no more than verifying that an interview took place, making a diagnosis, perhaps making a treatment plan, and writing rudimentary progress notes. Since there were no specific standards, good documentation was a matter of subjective opinion. Although clinical judgment will always be an extremely important part of understanding client behaviors, there must be a balance of incorporating universal procedures (e.g., *Diagnostic and Statistical Manual of Mental Disorders, Fourth Edition, Text Revision* (American Psychiatric Association, 2000) criteria, professional regulations, accreditation requirements) when documenting services. Insurance companies that paid for mental health services listed few or no documentation requirements to validate a diagnosis or the client's need for services. Clients receiving mental health services seldom knew their diagnosis or even if there was a treatment plan. Now, the client is an important part in formulating the treatment plan.

Today, in the age of professional accountability, clinical proficiency is necessary but not sufficient in providing mental health services. Third-party payers demand evidence that demonstrates both the need and effectiveness of mental health treatment. An insurance company or an accreditation agency does not interview a client to determine the effectiveness of services. (However, at times, outcomes surveys are sent to clients.) They rely on written documentation from the therapist. Therefore, if services are not properly documented, the most skillful therapist could appear on paper to be ineffective.

Some therapists often become upset when they see a client for a few sessions and then are required to request an authorization for additional services. If the therapist is not trained in documentation procedures, it is highly possible that further services could be denied even if the client highly needs treatment. The case manager reviewing the case has nothing to review other than the therapist's written evidence. When additional services are declined by a third-party reviewer, the rejection is more likely due to poor documentation, rather than a refusal to allow a needy client to receive treatment. The adage, "If it isn't written down, it doesn't exist," holds especially true for clinical documentation.

Today, no assumptions are made regarding the need for services, what took place in a session, or what progress has occurred. Auditors or reviewers do not attend therapy sessions to assess therapeutic effectiveness. The only effective means of communication therapists have with auditors is *written documentation*. This book provides examples and explanations of how to document the entire course of therapy.

WHAT WE "OUGHT TO DO" VERSUS WHAT WE WERE "TAUGHT TO DO"

Current documentation procedures required by third parties and accrediting agencies follow a medical model in which evidence of therapeutic effectiveness is based on observable and measurable client behaviors, rather than being solely based on intuition and insight. Undoubtedly, clinical intuition and insight are necessary clinical skills, but they are not sufficient for empirical documentation. Therapists may be trained from a wide range of theoretical perspectives, dealing with mild to severe degrees of client impairment and dysfunction. Therapists trained from a perspective emphasizing personal growth, increased insight, and clinical intuition are likely to be less comfortable learning documentation procedures from a medical model than those trained from a scientific-practitioner model. Their treatment is not the issue, for it may very well be as effective, or more effective, than other means of treatment. However, the issue is documentation of the effects of therapy, not the mode of therapy.

The criteria for the medical, also called the scientific-practitioner, model is based on diagnostic criteria found in the

DSM-IV-TR. This text will provide instruction in documentation that will be especially helpful to those whose training did not include a scientific-practitioner model. Typically third-party payers do not reimburse for services unless they are demonstrated as being medically necessary. Those who are trained to provide counseling that may be therapeutically helpful (e.g., personal growth counseling, relationship therapy), but is not medically necessary, are likely to find the material found in this text challenging to their basic assumptions but necessary for financial survival if they receive third-party payment. Documentation training will help ease the conflict of determining which services are covered by insurance.

MENTAL HEALTH GRADUATE TRAINING

Graduate school mental health training emphasizes theory and practice of psychotherapy. Training includes obtaining knowledge and understanding in a wide spectrum of clinical perspectives—assessment, interviewing, testing, diagnosis, ethics, statistics, research, and other areas. The numerous skills developed are quite time-consuming, providing little time for learning the mechanics of clinical practice, including documentation skills. Training in "treatment planning" typically involves planning a client's treatment but usually not how to write a treatment plan or document client behaviors during the treatment. Students are taught how to treat clients but not necessarily how to communicate in writing what will be conducted in therapy, what was conducted in therapy, and how to integrate the two.

It is clearly the intention of graduate school educators that students will learn documentation skills, but the training doesn't neatly fit into one particular graduate school course—and when considering the numerous required courses, there is usually no room for additional courses in most training programs. Even if documentation procedures are not taught specifically, it is usually assumed that students will be taught these procedures during their practicum or internship experiences. Oftentimes, though, documentation training does not take place here either because typically, in an internship, the graduate student sees clients pro bono or for a reduced fee, rather than through third-party payment; therefore, their documentation is not subject to third-party payer regulations. In addition, their clinical supervision focuses on the quality of therapy and case conceptualization skills, which, in themselves, are an arduous task to master. For these reasons, students' documentation skills are not typically scrutinized with the same rigor by their clinical supervisors as they would be by a third-party payer. Nevertheless, documentation training in graduate school is on the rise due to the realities in the field.

Third-Party Payers and Managed Care

Third-party payment to mental health providers is a relatively recent phenomenon. Lobbying on the part of mental health professionals and employers has led to the inclusion of mental health care in many health care insurance packages. However, more recently, mental health coverage has been increasingly restricted. There was a time in which, if a client's insurance policy covered mental health services, he or she could receive seemingly unlimited services from their provider of choice. Mental health providers simply filled out insurance forms and soon received payment. Not surprisingly, some people with minor diagnoses spent several years in counseling, with no review of therapeutic effectiveness. As a result, the cost of mental health benefits skyrocketed, and third-party payers had no choice but to find means to lower mental health costs to remain competitive and stay in business. Managed care, with its focus on cost containment, was the end result.

More than any other change agent, managed care has transformed the scope and nature of mental health services. Before managed care existed, it was possible to receive insurance benefits for nonmedically necessary counseling services. Costs skyrocketed. Thus, counseling services such as for personal growth, relationship therapy, and psychoeducational services are now not generally covered by insurance. This author is not negating the positive and life-changing effects of these types of counseling but is simply noting current third-party criteria for payment of mental health services.

Managed care has restricted the types of services available to those only viewed as medically necessary, and it requires that the therapist must, on an ongoing basis, demonstrate that additional services are necessary. When there is not sufficient evidence of a client's impairments being reduced as a result of mental health treatment, payment for services is discontinued. Without appropriate documentation, there is no means to gauge the effects of treatment. The medical model, or scientific-practitioner, model offered an effective means for achieving this requirement.

Although practitioners from different treatment modalities disagree about which therapeutic methods lead to effective change, documentation is theoretically neutral. Good documentation skills enable therapists from any school of thought to demonstrate the need for services and demonstrate therapeutic effectiveness. Therapists from all schools of thought can learn to document therapeutic progress and not worry about their insurance claims being rejected due to insufficient documentation.

Managed care's intent is to provide affordable services to clients. Therapists who learn thorough documentation procedures typically have no problem receiving payment for services and receiving authorization for continued services.

MEDICAL NECESSITY

The medical, or scientific-practitioner, model, which requires that services are *medically necessary* to qualify for third-party payment, has influenced current third-party reimbursement procedures for mental health services. Mental health services are considered medically necessary when the client is significantly impaired in areas such as social, occupational, educational, or other types of functioning, and without mental health services, the client is not likely to improve or return to premorbid functioning. Prior to adopting the medical necessity model, third-party payers paid for services when qualified clinicians diagnosed clients with a mental health disorder. This is still part of the process, but receiving a diagnosis alone is not sufficient to guarantee payment for services. A person who endorses a number of symptoms of, for example, Major Depressive Disorder, might be functioning adequately socially, occupationally, and in other areas. Simply experiencing some mental health symptoms may not fit the third party's criteria for coverage of mental health services. That is, services might be helpful but may not be necessary. One could say that there are two types of counseling services: those that are medically necessary (paid by insurance) and those that are not necessary (not paid by insurance) both of which are helpful to the client.

Criteria for diagnosing a mental health diagnosis have also been in transition. The typical procedure several years ago for making a diagnosis was simple endorsement of mental health symptoms that defined a diagnosis. For example, if a client endorses having a number of symptoms of depression, such as weight loss, low appetite, sadness, decreased concentration, and decreased sleep, it is likely that a diagnosis would be given in the past solely based on symptoms. However, simply endorsing symptoms is not enough because it does not imply the degree (i.e., mild to severe) of the symptoms or their effect on the client's functioning. Current diagnosis procedures must validate both the existence and degree of symptoms, plus demonstrate that there are resultant impairments as a result of the mental health disorder.

The degree to which symptoms affect the client's behavior and functioning is much more significant than acknowledging that symptoms exist. To qualify for treatment reimbursement, symptoms must be documented so that a third-party review can understand their impact on the client. Thus, clinicians must also learn to document the onset, frequency, antecedents, intensity, and duration of symptoms plus the resulting functional impairments when documenting.

MENTAL HEALTH CRITERIA

Some third-party payers provide vague criteria for reimbursement for mental health services, supplying few, if any, examples of what is expected in documentation. There are no clear statuary requirements, other than from state-funded Medicaid. Medicaid provider manuals range from a few pages to several hundred pages of regulations depending on the state. Some states that license mental health facilities periodically audit charts to monitor the quality of services. State licensure boards typically publish some guidelines for documentation, but not at the specificity of managed care or accrediting agencies.

Few widely accepted standards of documentation exist. Even

Comparison to Documentation in Other Fields

When someone has an auto accident and has insurance coverage to pay for the car being repaired, the insurance company will not accept a bill from the repair shop until evidence of what repairs took place is provided. Their methods of documentation may include photographs of the damage and a detailed list of services that are concordant with acceptable standards. Likewise, when a dentist performs services, X-rays are sent to the insurance company as evidence of the need for services. In the delivery of mental health services, it is not possible to take photographs or X-rays of the damage; therefore, we provide written documentation that follows the same general principles.

the standards from accreditation agencies (e.g., CARF, JCAHO), who publish extensive manuals of standards, there is room for subjective interpretation. This writer recalls a recent accreditation visit in which the auditors sent from the accreditation agency appeared to have difficulty agreeing on rating various charts.

Third-party payers have different specific requirements for reimbursement of services from state to state and company to company, but many of the guidelines are fairly consistent, such as:

1. Services must be medically or therapeutically necessary.
2. Services must be directed toward a diagnosable mental illness or disorder.
3. Services must be consistent with the diagnosis and degree of impairment.
4. There must be documentation of reasonable progress consistent with the treatment of the disorder.
5. The treatment plan must include specific discharge criteria written in behavioral terms.
6. Services must be specifically directed toward the diagnosis.
7. To receive continued services, there must be documented evidence of continued impairment.
8. The progress notes must clearly reflect the treatment plan goals and objectives.

Without such criteria, there is no clear means of documenting that the services being rendered are needed. Although third-party payers' specific regulations regarding forms, frequency of reports, and so forth may differ in some areas, the overall information requested is remarkably similar.

CRITERIA FOR CLINICAL SIGNIFICANCE

The *DSM-IV-TR* (APA, 2000) states:

> The definition of mental disorder in the introduction to DSM-IV-TR requires that there be clinically significant impairment or distress. To highlight the importance of considering this issue, the criteria sets for most disorders include a clinical significance criterion (usually worded ". . . causes clinically significant distress or impairment in

social, occupational, or other important areas of functioning.") This criterion helps establish the threshold for the diagnosis of a disorder in those situations in which the symptomatic presentation by itself (particularly in its milder forms) is not inherently pathological and may be encountered in individuals for whom a diagnosis of "mental disorder" would be inappropriate . . ." (p. 8).

The OFAID (of Aid) Procedure

The acronym *OFAID* is a helpful procedure that may be used throughout the course of therapy to help provide measurable evidence of client progresses. The information, additionally, helps confirm a diagnosis and demonstrate outcomes of treatment. The OFAID acronym stands for the following:

Onset:	Date or time period when symptoms began
Frequency:	How often symptoms occur
Antecedents:	Events or stressors leading to onset/exacerbation of symptoms
Intensity:	Severity of symptoms (e.g., Mild, Moderate, Severe, or 1–100)
Duration:	How long symptoms last

Example of Documentation with OFAID Procedure

Client with depression. Nicole states that she has been depressed for the past year since her child was removed from the home by social services (*onset*). She states that she feels depressed over 90% of the time (*frequency*). She becomes increasingly more depressed when she sees little children, which remind her of her child who is currently placed in foster care (*antecedents*). When asked about the level of her depression, she states that on a 1–100 scale it is usually around 85–90 (*intensity*). She further adds that during bouts of depression, she isolates herself in her room up to 10 hours per day (*duration*).

Client with panic attacks. Tyler began having panic attacks when he lost his job 6 months ago (*onset*). Currently, he has an average of three panic attacks per day (*frequency*). Panic attacks typically take place when he leaves the house, when the phone rings, or when someone comes to his door (*antecedents*). He describes the effects as severe, which he rates as a 95 on a scale of 1–100 (*intensity*). He states that his panic attacks last an average of 20 minutes (*duration*).

Use of the OFAID Procedure in Validating a Diagnosis

Although validating a diagnosis will be discussed in more detail in Chapter 5, a brief explanation of this procedure will be given at this time of validating a diagnosis with the OFAID procedure (see Table 2.1).

The *DSM-IV-TR* lists specific requirements that must be met in order to make a diagnosis. The specific types of requirements vary by diagnosis; however, the OFAID procedure is helpful in validating or providing supportive evidence that the diagnosis given to a client matches specific *DSM-IV-TR* criteria.

The *DSM-IV-TR* suggests it is possible for a person to experience symptoms of a disorder but not be diagnosed as such because symptoms are not severe enough. On the other hand, inadequate documentation can make clients appear to be less afflicted than they actually are. If medical necessity is not found to be evident due to insufficient or inadequate documentation, reimbursement will be denied. The following examples highlight incidents where medical necessity is not adequately documented:

TABLE 2.1
Example of Use of OFAID Procedure in Validating a Diagnosis of Major Depressive Disorder

DSM-IV-TR *criteria for diagnosis*	*Example of validation*
Depressive symptoms or lack of pleasure for at least 2 weeks	"Client has been depressed for the past 8 months." (*onset*)
Depressed most of the time	"Client states that she is depressed 5 or more days per week." (*frequency* and *duration*)
	No *DSM-IV-TR* requirement for antecedents for this diagnosis
Qualifiers of *Mild, Moderate, Severe,* and other descriptors	"Level of depression is Severe, due to significant impairments socially and occupationally." (*intensity*)

Note: Not every facet of OFAID is required in this case.

- *Poorly Documented Example:* "The client is depressed, withdrawn, suffers from lack of sleep and fatigue, feels anxious, and has feelings of confusion."

Specific Problems in the Documentation: This statement does not provide adequate documentation for a diagnosis because it lists only symptoms. Impairments are not validated. It is possible that the client is functioning adequately because the severity of symptoms is minimal.

A normal life stressor could lead to these symptoms. People at times experience some degree of these symptoms and are not considered psychopathological. For example, if a person fails an important college exam, it is possible that the person, for a few days, could feel down, avoid others, lose some sleep, and feel tired. These symptoms, on paper, might look like a Depressive Disorder, but when considering other factors, such as duration and intensity of symptoms, they appear to be a normal reaction to a normal life stressor. The preceding symptoms are expected, given the situation.

Properly Documented Example: "The client meets criteria for major depression as evidenced by feeling depressed most of the time for the past two months, withdrawing from almost all people, daily suicidal ideations, sleeping less than three hours per night, physical and mental fatigue, and increased worrying. There is resulting educational and social impairment in that he has not attended college classes in over one month and usually stays in his room by himself, avoiding friends and family."

- *Poorly Documented Example:* "The client has panic attacks."

Specific Problems in the Documentation: This statement also does not provide enough information to warrant a diagnosis of a mental disorder. The label "panic attacks" could be explained using the OFAID procedure to provide a clearer picture of the history and level of symptomology. Many people have had at least one panic attack in their lives, but it does not constitute a Panic Disorder. Others have frequent, debilitating panic attacks causing significant dysfunction that interferes with a wide array of daily activities. The main problem with this statement is that it could apply to someone with panic attacks of any degree, whether very mild or severe.

Properly Documented Example: "The client has experienced Panic Disorder without Agoraphobia. Symptoms last at least thirty minutes, and have occurred at least twice per day for the past year.

Symptoms included palpitations, hot flashes, sweating, chest pains, dizziness, trembling, and fleeing the situation. During the past three months, panic attacks have increased in duration and intensity, resulting in avoiding any new or stressful situations and leaving work early approximately three to four times per week. He has gone to the emergency room three times in the past month, believing that he was going to die."

• *Poorly Documented Example:* "The client is having trouble coping with a recent divorce and death of a loved one."

Specific Problems in the Documentation: This statement does not justify the need for treatment. These are normal life stressors or events that many people experience. There is no evidence of abnormal impairments or a need for mental health services. It is expected that a person would have difficulty coping with a recent divorce and the death of a loved one, but there is no documented evidence of a mental health disorder. Although mental health counseling might be needed, there is no supporting evidence.

Properly Documented Example: "The client is experiencing an Adjustment Disorder with Depressed Mood as evidenced by increased depression, withdrawal, and difficulties coping. Symptoms have occurred since the onset of two major stressors in the past three months, including the death of his mother and his divorce. Affective impairment is noted as evidenced by feeling dysphoric most of the time and having difficulties feeling motivated to work, shop, or resume usual activities. Concerns include crying several times per day, missing work at least twice per week, and avoiding all social supports."

• *Poorly Documented Example:* "The client goes to work only one or two days per week, has no friends, and has not phoned any family members for more than two months."

Specific Problems in the Documentation: In this case, functional impairments may exist, but no mental disorder is documented. The impairment must be the result of a mental disorder to demonstrate medical necessity for receiving mental health treatment. Otherwise, services other than mental health may be needed.

The documentation also does not indicate whether these behaviors represent a significant change in functioning or if the client simply chooses to work temporary jobs sporadically and prefers to be alone. One cannot assume psychopathology based on a lifestyle that is not mainstream.

Properly Documented Example: "The client has felt depressed for the past three weeks as evidenced by suicidal ideations, feeling hopeless and worthless, and excessive eating. There is resulting affective, cognitive, educational, and physical impairment as evidenced by constant fatigue, missing school 50% of the time from lack of sleep (average three hours per night), decreased concentration (unable to comprehend after reading more than three to four minutes at a time), weight gain of 12 pounds in past three weeks, and increased negative self-statements noted by others."

Figure 2.1 provides a helpful format to use when documenting a client's symptoms and resulting impairments or dysfunctions. Documentation procedures that state only whether symptoms exist can be compared to stating that an automobile tire is low on air. Most automobile tires at some time are low on air. This may be because the automobile has hit a bump, cold weather, or even due to normal wear. Just because a tire is low on air does not always mean the driver cannot drive the car. The severity of the problem depends, in part, on how low on air the tire is. Other descriptors, such as how long there has been trouble with the tire losing air, how often it must be filled up, and the condition of the tire, will help you make a more informed decision about whether to continue driving the car or to take it in for service. Likewise, listing mental health symptoms alone does not provide enough specific information to make a diagnosis or plan treatment.

Figure 2.2 illustrates the difference between simply listing a client's symptoms and documenting the impacts of those symptoms by adding qualifiers to demarcate additional dimensions of impairment. Profile 1 represents two clients appearing to suffer from the same problem. Notice the difference, however, when further descriptors are added in Profile 2.

Adding the descriptors of the OFAID procedure provides evi-

FIGURE 2.1
Suggested Format for Documenting Client Symptoms and Functional Impairments

The client has been experiencing _____*(problem area)*_____ for the past _*(time span)*_
as evidenced by _____*(list of symptoms that are concordant with DSM-IV)*_____,
resulting in _____*(specific areas of impairment)*_____ impairment(s) as evidenced by
(specific examples of functional impairments).

FIGURE 2.2
Two Profiles of Clients Presenting with Major Depression

Profile 1 Listing Symptoms Only	
Client A	**Client B**
Depressed mood	Depressed mood
Social withdrawal	Social withdrawal
Suicidal ideations	Suicidal ideations
Lack of pleasure	Lack of pleasure
Poor concentration	Poor concentration
Weight gain	Weight gain

Profile 2   Listing Additional Descriptors for Clients A and B Documents Difference in Diagnosis and Medical Necessity

Client A		**Client B**
Onset:	4 years ago	12 years ago
Frequency:	2 episodes since onset	2–3 episodes/year (cycling)
Duration:	Episodes last ≤ 2 weeks	Episodes last 30–45 days
Severity:	Mild	Severe, occasional psychotic features
Extent of impaired function:	Sometimes late for work	Recently fired from job, 8 job losses,
	No job losses	no friends, 4 suicide attempts,
	Sometimes avoid friends	6 hospitalizations for depression,
	No hospitalizations	currently in bankruptcy, emerging panic symptoms, gained 35 lbs.
	Gained 10 lbs. in past 6 months	in past 6 months

dence that Client B is more severely impaired than Client A. Documentation procedures that address only symptomology miss this important distinction. For this reason, it is difficult to make a clear diagnosis when only symptoms are described. Likewise, it is difficult to convince third-party payers that a diagnosis (or treatment) is warranted when only symptoms are documented.

In addition, when documentation of specific functional or behavioral impairment is lacking, there is meager evidence to use in determining the type and number of services most appropriate for the client. The *DSM-IV-TR* (APA, 2000) states, "Making a DSM-IV diagnosis is only the first step in a comprehensive evaluation. To formulate an adequate treatment plan, the clinician will invariably require considerable additional information about the person being evaluated beyond that required to make a DSM-IV diagnosis" (p. xxxv).

Appropriate documentation for diagnosis, treatment planning, and reimbursement requires specifying the degree to which symptoms are impairing various areas of the client's functioning. Current standards in documentation incorporate the level of functional impairment as the measurement standard of the effects of mental illness symptoms. Incorporating impairments and dysfunctions presents a clearer picture of a client's mental status. Also, decisions regarding the medical necessity of treatment are more clearly communicated, and treatment planning may be written and understood more clearly.

FUNCTIONAL IMPAIRMENTS

Functional impairments are significant dysfunctions in daily living, impacting affective, cognitive, occupational, social, or other functioning for which the client needs mental health services (i.e., medical necessity is demonstrated) to adequately return to normal or previous levels of functioning. In other words, without such services, the client is likely to remain dysfunctional. For example, a currently depressed person might have a history of going to work and working productively 5 days per week. Since the onset of depression, however, the client has been attending work only 2 to 3 days per week, resulting in significantly decreased production, and is in jeopardy of termination. This same client may also be experiencing increased social withdrawal and avoiding previous friends, thereby cutting off potential social supports. Areas of impairment for this client are described as *occupational* and *social*. Other areas of impairment due to depression could exist also, including physical, affective, cognitive impairments, and any other aspect in which a person's activities of daily living are restricted due to a mental disorder. Figure 2.3 provides various examples of functional impairments.

Because current documentation guidelines (medical model) require providing observable and measurable evidence of changes in functional impairments resulting from treatment, the diagnostic interview should include obtaining baseline measures of the client's degree of functional impairment.

FIGURE 2.3
Examples of Functional Impairments

Occupational	"Work production for the client has decreased by more than 75% since the death of his spouse, resulting in potential termination if quota is not met by July 10th."
Academic	"Recent school reports indicate that client is angry at classmates, teachers, and family members almost all of the time making it difficult to concentrate on academics. Grades have dropped two letter grades in the past two terms."
Social	"Client has not left her house nor contacted any family members in the past five months, since panic attacks began. Previously client was highly involved socially and with her family."
	"Client is ostracized by classmates due to hyperactivity and immature behaviors on the playground. Frustration, aggressive outbursts, and temper tantrums have increased."
Affective	"Client reports significant sadness, boredom, and grief, resulting in increased suicidal threats."
Physical	"Client reports inability to perform usual activities of daily living, extreme fatigue, increased headaches, loss of 40 lbs. due to low appetite, and dizziness since losing his job."
Combinations	"Client's mother indicates that he is failing in school, has lost all of his friends, has been fired from his job, and has been arrested for marijuana possession for the third time. Before he was injured in the auto accident he received As and Bs in school, seldom missed work, and had no history of drug or alcohol use."

ASSESSMENT PROCEDURES

The initial diagnostic session is the backbone of clinical assessment. All other documentation is based on this initial information. Although new information is provided regularly throughout treatment, it is the foundation of treatment. Assessment procedures provide a clinical history and current snapshot of the purpose for which services are needed. Several aspects of the client's life are reviewed and subsequently integrated in a diagnostic summary that considers a full range of function status. Without the assessment there would be no identification of client strengths, weaknesses, preferences; thus, no information would be available to provide an accurate treatment plan. Figure 2.4 lists CARF requirements for the initial assessment.

FIGURE 2.4
Overview of CARF (2004) Standards for Assessment

1. The organization continuously conducts assessments or obtains information for each person served:
   a. In a manner that is respectful and considerate of that person's specific needs.
   b. That identifies the expectations of the person served.
   c. That provides for the use of assistive technology or resources, as needed, in the assessment process.
   d. That is responsive to the changing needs of the person served.
   e. That includes provisions for communicating the results of the assessment to:
      (1) Personnel.
      (2) The person served.
      (3) Appropriate others.
   f. That provides the basis for legally required notification, when applicable.

2. Assessments are conducted by qualified personnel:
   a. Knowledgeable to assess the specific needs of the persons served.
   b. Trained in the use of applicable tools.

3. The assessments include information obtained from:
   a. The person served.
   b. Family members, when applicable or permitted.
   c. Friends or peers, when appropriate and permitted.
   d. Other appropriate and permitted collateral sources.

4. The primary assessment gathers sufficient information to develop an individualized, person-centered plan for each person served, including information about the person's:
   a. Personal strengths
   b. Individual needs.
   c. Abilities and interests.
   d. Preferences.
   e. Presenting problems.
   f. Urgent needs, including suicide risk.
   g. Previous behavioral health services, including:
      (1) Diagnostic information.
      (2) Treatment information.
      (3) Efficacy of current or previously used medications.
   h. Physical health history and current status.
   i. Diagnosis(es).

FIGURE 2.4 (Continued)

---

j. Mental status.

k. Current level of functioning.

l. Pertinent current and historical life situation information, including his or her:

    (1) Age.

    (2) Gender.

    (3) Employment history.

    (4) Legal involvement.

    (5) Family history.

    (6) History of abuse.

    (7) Relationships, including natural supports.

m. Issues important to the person served.

n. Use of alcohol, tobacco, and/or other drugs.

o. Need for, and availability of, social supports.

p. Risk-taking behaviors.

q. Level of educational functioning.

r. Advance directives, when applicable.

s. Medication use profile.

t. Medication allergies or adverse reactions to medications.

u. Adjustments to disabilities/disorders.

5. The primary assessment:

    a. Is conducted within specific time frames.

    b. Results in the preparation of an interpretive summary that is:

        (1) Based on the assessment data.

        (2) Used in the development of the treatment plan.

        (3) Identifies any co-occurring disabilities/disorders that should be addressed in the development of the individual plan.

Source: Used by permission of the Behavioral Health Standards Manual. Commission on Accreditation of Rehabilitation Facilities. Copyright 2004.

TREATMENT PLANNING

Although the collection of clinical information is ongoing, the information gathered in the initial diagnostic assessment is most crucial because it directly affects the treatment plan, progress notes, and subsequent reports. The treatment plan is based on the diagnostic assessment. All information written in the treatment plan must correspond to the assessment and information gathered in subsequent sessions. That is, targeted issues for treatment should be carefully examined in the intake and subsequent sessions, rather than simply appearing in the treatment plan without written justification that a need for treatment exists.

The treatment plan is a dynamic document that is subject to revisions as treatment progresses and more information is learned about the client. A well-formed treatment plan is crucial to ensuring reimbursement for services because it provides a blueprint of therapy. Like a teacher's lesson plan, it outlines the recipient's needs, functioning level, and describes in a step-by-step manner how to meet the intended goals via specific objectives. Likewise, properly written progress notes are important because they are the sole source of documentation that treatment plan goals and objectives are being met.

THE FINANCIAL IMPACT OF CLINICAL DOCUMENTATION

In the not-so-distant past, third-party reimbursement for mental health services was virtually guaranteed. Today, however, the quality of documentation directly affects the financial status of the clinic and therapist. The effect of an audit can result, and often has resulted, in therapists facing thousands of dollars in financial penalties to third parties when client charts are not in compliance with accepted standards. Many clinics have gone bankrupt because they were unable to return funds to an insurance company after an audit. Keep in mind that paybacks do not always indicate that treatment was unwarranted or that a therapist was unscrupulous. It is possible that the therapist can provide appropriate treatment but be penalized financially due to insufficient documentation.

One common auditing procedure incorporated by third-party payers is to audit a set number of charts and use that as the basis for determining what percentage of files at the clinic are not in compliance with documentation procedures. For example, if 100 charts are audited and 20 are determined not to demonstrate medical necessity for services, the insurance company may determine that 20% of all monies it paid to the clinic during the audit period (often 1 to 3 years) must be paid back. In this case, if a clinic employs five therapists who each see an average of 10 patients from the auditor's insurance company per week, the total number of visits would look like this:

$$
\begin{array}{rl}
5 & \text{Therapists} \\
\times\ 10 & \text{Clients per week (from the insurance provider} \\
& \text{conducting the audit)} \\
\times\ 52 & \text{Weeks per year} \\
\underline{\times\ \ \ 3} & \text{Years (audit period)} \\
7{,}800 & \text{Client visits reimbursed by the insurance provider}
\end{array}
$$

This results in a total of 7,800 client visits in the 3-year period. If the insurance company reimbursed the clinic $60 per visit, the total payment to the clinic in the 3-year period would be $468,000. An audit resulting in 20% noncompliance would suggest a 20% payback totaling $93,600 plus interest! One therapist (of the five), at this rate, would owe the insurance company $18,200 for seeing only 10 clients per week from one paying source! Most therapists would have tremendous difficulty paying back such an audit. If the clinic is footing the bill, two usual payback procedures are for the insurance company to deduct payment from its future reimbursements to the clinic or for the clinic to pay back a set amount monthly. Either procedure makes it difficult to meet payroll until the amount is paid off (which often is the time for another audit).

In the event that a clinic will face an audit, there should be clear contractual or employment contract provisions between the clinic and its therapists to determine who is responsible for audit paybacks. When therapists are paid based on a commission of fees received, contracts generally state that the clinician will pay back the income received from the specific files under audit. For example, if the clinician is paid 55% of money received for services, his or her payback amount would be 55% of the total payback for his or her portion of the audit. The procedure is more difficult for clinics that pay therapists salaries because, in most cases, the clinic bears the brunt of the entire payback. Fortunately, clear and thorough documentation drastically reduces the possibility of making paybacks to third parties.

Accurate documentation procedures not only help a clinic remain in business but also provide for clinical and ethical responsibility. They aid in accurate diagnosis, treatment planning, continued demonstration of need for services, and validating the effects of therapy. Documentation skills do not add to the level of paperwork in the therapeutic process. On the contrary, when good documentation procedures are adopted, the time needed to accurately chart a case decreases.

LEGAL ISSUES IN DOCUMENTATION

A major focus in the study of litigation in mental health malpractice has been examining psychological records (Fulero & Wilbert, 1988). Over- and underdocumentation poses different sets of problems. Documenting everything that takes place in treatment may violate the client's confidentiality in areas that are not necessary to document therapeutically, whereas underdocumenting may fail to document that specific services are taking place. In a 1988 study, Fulero and Wilbert found that more than 50% of therapists surveyed withheld nothing in their patients' records. Other therapists endorsed withholding information in patients' records regarding (a) speculations or opinions, (b) others' names, (c) keep no or minimal records anyway, (d) anything damaging, (e) highly personal information, (f) infidelity, (g) sexual preference or behavior, (h) process notes, (i) diagnostic labels, (j) criminal behaviors, and others.

Soisson, VandeCreek, and Knapp (1987) reviewed cases in which records influenced the outcomes of malpractice suits. They noted that in a malpractice claim, the plaintiff must demonstrate that:

1. The practitioner (defendant) owed a duty to the client (plaintiff) based on an established therapeutic relationship.
2. The quality of care provided by the practitioner fell below the standard of care expected of the average practitioner.
3. The patient suffered or caused harm or injury.
4. The practitioner's dereliction of duty was the direct cause of harm or injury (Cohen, 1979).

The most common grounds for malpractice are identified as:

1. Unauthorized release of information,
2. Negligent treatment of suicidal or aggressive patients,
3. Sexual relations between patient and therapist,
4. Failure to diagnose adequately, and
5. Improper hospitalization of a patient.

In each of these examples, thorough clinical documentation is crucial in the psychotherapist's defense. Specific information in the patient's record may demonstrate that effective therapeutic principles were followed, but the client did not comply or was not honest in the clinical presentation.

In cases of suicide, the practitioner or agency has not been held legally responsible when records indicate that adequate assessment and treatment procedures were conducted (*Dalton v. State,* 1970; *Johnson v. United States,* 1976). Without adequate documentation, the therapist has been held accountable in litigation. Slovenko (1979) describes an inadequate record as an indicative of poor care. Likewise, adequate records, but with poor follow-up of the clinical observations, may put the therapist in jeopardy.

Gutheil and Appelbaum (1982) state that clinical records should be written from the perspective of future readers. Soisson et al. (1987) suggest that in the case of a suicidal client, documentation should include an assessment of the risk, options considered for the prevention of suicide, and possible treatments (including advantages and disadvantages).

The treatment process is a series of systematic procedures in which most aspects of the client's life are examined in order to rule out specific areas of impairment that might otherwise be overlooked. The biopsychosocial assessment is designed to integrate past and present behaviors. It is the first clinical procedure in the assessment and treatment process.

HIGHLIGHTS
of Chapter 2

★ Clinical skills, in themselves, are not sufficient to obtain extended services for clients when third-party payers are involved. Documentation skills are needed to demonstrate accountability.

★ Graduate school training in mental health services has often assumed that documentation skills are being learned at internship sites, but this may not be the case.

★ Although any level of counseling may be helpful to clients, third-party reimbursement generally requires that mental health services be medically necessary for services to be reimbursed.

* In mental health, medical necessity is demonstrated by the existence of a mental health disorder resulting in significant functional impairments, which, without treatment, the client is not likely to improve or return to premorbid functioning in a timely manner.

* Without documentation of functional impairments, it is difficult to assess the need for mental health services.

* Indicators such as onset, frequency, antecedents, intensity, and duration (OFAID procedure) significantly increase the specificity of documentation of the diagnosis, symptoms, and impairments.

* Documentation skills can improve with adequate training and simplified procedures.

* Mental health services from any school of thought can be documented in measurable and behavioral terms.

* Poor documentation significantly increases a clinician's chances of being held liable in litigation.

* Therapists are encouraged to conduct therapy from their choice of schools of thought, but documentation procedures are written according to a medical model in behavioral terms (scientific-practitioner).

QUESTIONS

1. When third-party payment is involved, clinical skills are necessary for _____, while documentation skills are necessary for _____.

   (a) therapeutic progress, termination of services.

   (b) rapport, therapeutic progress.

   (c) therapeutic progress, continuation of services.

   (d) continuation of services, termination of services.

2. Stringent documentation requirements are considered important at this time because it helps

   (a) control mental health costs.

   (b) demonstrate the need for services.

   (c) provide specific diagnostic information.

   (d) all of these.

3. Which of the following statements best describes the concept of *medical necessity?*

    (a) Without mental health services, the client will likely remain dysfunctional.

    (b) Without mental health services, the client could develop medical problems.

    (c) Services are necessary because of the client's current medical condition.

    (d) Services are necessary to enhance the client's self-concept.

4. What is the primary purpose of the OFAID procedure?

    (a) to aid the client in therapy.

    (b) to obtain objective information about client behaviors.

    (c) to prove that a client needs services.

    (d) to provide information beyond the requirements of the *DSM-IV-TR.*

5. Which of the following best represents a functional impairment?

    (a) The client's symptoms include low appetite, poor sleep, worrying, frustration, and low self-esteem.

    (b) The client doesn't feel as happy as in the past and therefore desires counseling.

    (c) The client is in danger of losing another job due to excessive absences due to depression.

    (d) The client quit his job due to boredom. He is now looking for a job but is unemployed.

6. The potential consequences of lack of documentation in cases such as suicide or homicide could lead to

    (a) loss of licensure.

    (b) significant ethical and legal issues.

    (c) financial consequences.

    (d) all of these.

Answers: 1. c; 2. d; 3. a; 4. b; 5. c; 6. d

3

The Biopsychosocial Assessment

The biopsychosocial assessment provides background information regarding several areas of the client's functioning. The bulk of the information is obtained through questioning in the initial interview and through forms the client fills out. Additions and revisions are made throughout treatment. Information covered includes biological (or physical), psychological, and social. Biological information includes information about the client's family, development, education, employment, legal, and other medical history. Psychological information focuses on previous and current psychological status and treatment. Social information includes the client's social supports and stressors.

Information regarding both the client's strengths and weaknesses should be collected for each aspect of the biopsychosocial assessment. Information about the client's strengths is helpful in treatment by incorporating positive aspects in the client's environment. For example, if the client has a supportive social network, treatment might include incorporating these people. Documenting and incorporating weakness is important in selecting what type(s) of treatment would be most suitable for the client.

General demographic information, such as number of years of schooling, may be obtained in preinterview questionnaires. The clinician reviews this information for clinical significance and incorporates it into the assessment when helpful. If the information suggests therapeutic significance, it may be incorporated in the treatment plan.

It is important to avoid redundancy in the primary information gathering period. If clients provide information prior to the initial interview, do not ask them for the same information in the interview unless it is being expanded upon. In such cases, nothing new is learned and time is wasted if the same questions are asked in presession questionnaires, phone screenings, and in the diagnostic assessment interview. Moreover, the client is likely to become frustrated if the initial phone screening, a presession questionnaire, and the clinician solicit the same information. Rather, each method of information gathering should integrate and expand on data already collected. For example, instead of asking about a client's marital status at each stage of information gathering, the initial phone screening might determine the marital status, a presession questionnaire might identify relationship issues, and the clinician might probe stressors, strengths, and dynamics of the relationship (if applicable) in the diagnostic interview.

The diagnostic assessment is *not* intended to be a counseling session. Focusing on counseling during the initial interview may be counterproductive because the time is needed to collect discrete types of information. However, a clinician who skillfully conducts the diagnostic interview in both an empathic and professional manner can assure clients that they are understood and allow them to leave the interview ready for treatment. Thus, the diagnostic session may ultimately have the effects of a productive counseling session even though no therapy was offered. After a successful interview a client feels understood.

Each individual piece of information collected in the biopsychosocial assessment in itself may not seem significant but, when taken together, helps present a clear clinical picture of the client. At this point, the therapist is no longer dealing with unrelated data but with the whole person in the realm of his or her past and present environment.

CONDUCTING THE BIOPSYCHOSOCIAL ASSESSMENT

Prior to conducting the initial interview, it is necessary to obtain the client's *informed consent*. The therapist should begin by informing the client of the purpose of the interview and how results will be disseminated. Written statements in the initial interview such as, "The client acknowledges and understands the benefits and risks of providing the information requested in this evaluation and has agreed to allow results to be shared with . . ." document informed consent. Some clinicians have the client sign that they have had the information explained to them. A summary of HIPAA guidelines for dissemination of information are found in Appendix C.

All of the information should be reviewed to produce a diagnosis and subsequent treatment plan. Some clinicians prefer to mail all preinterview questionnaires to clients and ask them to fill them out prior to the first meeting. Others ask the client to come early to the initial interview to fill out the questionnaires.

Using preformatted questionnaires can save time for the clinician. For example, Figures 3.1 and 3.2 follow similar formats that allow the clinician to more easily access information when writing reports and treatment plans and reviewing cases. Figure 3.1 provides an example of a client personal history form. Figure 3.2, an example of an initial intake, which also includes biopsychosocial information, is a report the therapist fills out after collecting sufficient information from the client. Some clinicians do not formally conduct a biopsychosocial assessment but prefer a structured or unstructured initial interview. There are no universally accepted formats for documenting a biopsychosocial assessment, but several exist commercially and in various texts. *The Clinical Documentation Sourcebook,* third edition (Wiger, 2005) provides mental health forms, examples of how to effectively fill them out, and a computer disk to aid in the documentation process.

There are three commonly accepted steps for conducting a biopsychosocial assessment:

1. Determining the presenting problem,
2. Recording the history, and
3. Assessing client strengths and limitations.

After the information is gathered, it should be written up in a psychological report of the problem.

STEP ONE: Presenting Problem (Signs and Symptoms)

The presenting problem is the client's description of the problem rather than the clinician's opinion or diagnostic statements. It is recorded in the section of the psychological report labeled "Signs and Symptoms." Although the terms *signs* and *symptoms* are generally combined or used synonymously, the *DSM-IV-TR* (APA, 2000) defines signs as "an objective manifestation of pathological condition. Signs are observed by the examiner rather than reported by the affected individual" (p. 827), whereas symptoms are defined as

FIGURE 3.1
Personal History Form

Adult Personal History Form

Case No. _053983D_

Client's Name __John Doe__   Date __5-3-05__

Gender __F ✔M__   Date of Birth __2-15-60__   Age __45__

Form completed by (if someone other than client)_____

Address __34567 Main Street__

City __Longview__   State __CA__   Zip __99999__

Phone (Home) __(555)-555-1213__   (Work) __(555) 555-1211__   ext. __9876__

IF YOU NEED ANY MORE SPACE FOR ANY OF THE FOLLOWING QUESTIONS PLEASE USE THE BACK OF THE SHEET

Primary reason(s) for seeking services: __Addictive behavors   __Alcohol/drugs
__Anger management   __Anxiety   __Coping   ✔Depression
__Eating disorder   __Fear/phobias   __Mental confusion   __Sexual concerns
__Sleeping problems   __Other mental health concerns (specify)_____

FAMILY INFORMATION

Relationship	Name	Age	Living Yes	Living No	Living with you Yes	Living with you No
Mother	Debra Doe	X		✔		✔
Father	Robert Doe	X		✔		✔
Spouse	None (1-Deceased 2-Divorced)		①✔	②✔		✔
Children	Cynthia Doe	16	✔			✔
	Victoria Doe	13	✔			✔

Significant Others (Brothers, Sisters, Grandparents, Step-relatives, Half-relatives. Please specify relationship.)

Relationship	Name	Age	Living Yes	Living No	Living with you Yes	Living with you No
Brother	Raymond Doe	48	✔			✔

FIGURE 3.1 (Continued)

Marital Status   (more than one answer may apply)

__Single

__Divorce in process
Length of time_____

__Unmarried, living together
Length of time_____

__Legally married
Length of time_____

__Separated
Length of time_____

✓Divorced
Length of time **4 yrs.**

✓Widowed
Length of time **10 mos.**

__Annulment
Length of time_____

Total number of marriages ____

Assessment of Current Relationship (if applicable)   __Good   __Fair   ✓Poor **with ex-wife**

Parental Information
✓Parents legally married **(now deceased)**
__Parents have even been separated
__Parents ever divorced

__Mother remarried: Number of times_____
__Father remarried: Number of times_____

Special curcumstances (e.g. raised by person other than parents, information about spouse/children not living with you, etc.)
_____
_____

DEVELOPMENT

Are there special, unusual, or traumatic circumstances that affected your development: ✓No   __Yes
If Yes, which type(s) of child abuse? __Sexual ✓Physical __Verbal.   Abuse was as __Victim __Perpetrator
Other childhood issues: __Neglect __Inadequate nutrition   __Other (specify)_____
Comments re: Childhood development **My father often beat me up when I was a teenager**
_____
_____

SOCIAL RELATIONSHIPS

Check how you generally get along with other people: (check all which apply)

✓Affectionate
✓Friendly
__Other (specify)_____

__Aggressive
__Leader

__Avoidant
__Outgoing

__Fight/argue often
✓Shy/withdrawn

__Follower
__Submissive

Sexual Orientation: **heterosexual**   Comments:_____

Sexual Dysfunctions? ✓No   __Yes (describe)_____

Any current or history of being as sexual perpetrator? ✓No   __Yes (describe)_____

CULTURAL / ETHNIC

From which cultural or ethinic group, if any, do you belong? **WASP**_____
Are you experiencing any problems due to culturual or ethnic issues? ✓No   __Yes (describe)_____

Other cultural / ethnic information:_____
_____

Page 2

(continued)

FIGURE 3.1 (Continued)

SPIRITUAL / RELIGIOUS

How important to you are spiritual matters? __Not __Little __Moderate ✓Much
Are you affiliated with a spiritual or religious group? ✓No __Yes (describe)_____
Were you raised within a spiritual or religious group? __No ✓Yes (describe) **very strict**
Would you like your spiritual/religious beliefs incorporated into the counseling? __No ✓Yes (describe) **I would like honest, ethical practices.**

LEGAL

Current Status

Are you involved in any active cases (traffic, civil, criminal)? __No ✓Yes
If Yes, please describe and indicate the court and hearing/trial dates and charges_____
Child support hearing in two weeks

Are you presently on probation or parole? ✓No __Yes
If Yes, please describe_____

Past History

Traffic violations	__No ✓Yes		DWI, DUI, etc.	✓No __Yes
Criminal involvement	✓No __Yes		Civil involvement	✓No __Yes

If you responded Yes to any of the above, please fill in the following information.

Charges	Date	Where (city)	Results
Speeding 45 in a 30	1985	Cambridge	Paid Fine

EDUCATIONAL

Fill in all that apply   Years of education __12__   Currently enrolled in school ✓No __Yes

✓High School grad/GED   __Vocational: Number of years____   Graduated __No __Yes   Major____
    __College: Number of years____   Graduated __No __Yes   Major____
    __Graduate: Number of years____   Graduated __No __Yes   Major____

Other training_____

Special circumstances (e.g. learning disabilities, gifted, etc.) **Average grades when in school**

EMPLOYMENT

Begin with most recent job, list job history:

Employer	Dates	Title	Reason left the job	How often miss work?
4M	1987-Present	Miller		lately 2days/wk
Stanford's	1984-1987	Laborer	new Job	seldom
Mengers	1979-1984	Laborer	new Job	seldom
Pollies	1975-1979	Sales	new Job	seldom

Currently: ✓FT __PT __Temp __Laid-off __Disabled __Retired __Social Security __Student
__Other (describe)_____

FIGURE 3.1 (Continued)

MILITARY

Military experience? __No ✓Yes Combat experience? ✓No __Yes Where?_____

Branch **Army**_____   Discharge date ___**1975**_____

Date drafted_____   Type of discharge **honorable**_____

Date enlisted __**1971**_____   Rank at discharge **Sargeant**_____

LEISURE / RECREATIONAL

Describe special areas of interest or hobbies (e.g., art, books, crafts, physical fitness, sports, outdoor activities, church activities, walking, exercising, diet/health, hunting, fishing, bowling, traveling, etc.)

Activity	How often now?	How often in the past?
Sports events	none	weekly
outdoor activities	seldom	weekly

MEDICAL / PHYSICAL HEALTH

Check all that apply and describe below:

__AIDS	__Constipation	__Hepatitis	__Sore throat
__Alcoholism	__Chicken Pox	__High blood pressure	__Scarlet Fever
__Abdominal pain	__Dental problems	__Kidney problems	__Sinusitis
__Abortion	__Diabetes	__Measles	__Small Pox
__Allergies	__Diarrhea	__Mononucleosis	__Stroke
__Anemia	__Dizziness	__Mumps	__Sexual problems
__Appendicitis	__Drug abuse	__Menstrual pain	__Tonsillitis
__Arthritis	__Epilepsy	__Miscarriages	__Tuberculosis
__Asthma	__Ear infections	__Neurological disorders	__Toothache
__Bronchitis	__Eating problems	__Nausea	__Thyroid problems
__Bed wetting	__Fainting	__Nose bleeds	__Vision problems
__Cancer	✓Fatigue	__Pneumonia	__Vomiting
__Chest pain	__Frequent urination	__Rheumatic Fever	__Whooping cough
__Chronic pain	__Headaches	__SexuallyTransmitted Diseases	__Other (describe)
__Colds/Coughs	__Hearing problems	__Sleeping disorders	

List any current health concerns __**low energy**_____

List any recent health or physical changes_____

Nutrition

Meal	How often (times per week)	Typical Foods Eaten	Typical amount eaten	Comments
Breakfast	**7** / week	cold cereal	__No __Low ✓Med __High	
Lunch	**6** / week	Soup-sandwich	__No __Low __Med ✓High	
Dinner	**7** / week	meat-potatoes-veg	__No __Low __Med ✓High	
Snacks	**20** / week	Junk food	__No __Low __Med ✓High	high appetite

Current Prescribed Medications	Dose	Dates	Purpose	Side Effects
None				

Current Over-the-counter Med's	Dose	Dates	Purpose	Side Effects
None				

Page 4

(continued)

FIGURE 3.1 (Continued)

Are you allergic to any medications or drugs? ✓ No __ Yes (describe)_____

	Date	Reason	Results
Last physical exam	2003	regular check-up	good health
Last doctor's visit	1999	strep throat	given antibiotic - OK
Last dental exam	2004	regular check-up	no problems
Most recent surgery	none		
Other surgery	none		
Upcoming surgery	none		

Family history of medical problems _Mother had thyroid condition._____

Please check if there have been any recent changes in the following
__Sleep patterns   ✓Eating patterns   __Behavior   ✓Energy level
__Physical activity level   __General disposition   ✓Weight   __Nervousness / tension
Describe changes in areas in which you checked above _Gaining weight from overeating and underactivity. Low energy: Don't feel like doing things._

CHEMICAL USE HISTORY

	Method of use and amount	Frequency of use	Age of first use	Age of last use	Used in last 48 hours		Used in last 30 days	
					Yes	No	Yes	No
Alcohol	lite social drinking	Rare	21	45		✓		✓
Barbiturates								
Valium/Librium								
Cocaine/Crack								
Heroin/Opiates								
Marijuana								
PCP/LSD/Mescaline								
Inhalants								
Caffeine								
Nicotine								
Over the counter								
Prescription drugs								
Other drugs								

Substance of preference

1. _None_____   3. _____

2. _____   4. _____

FIGURE 3.1 (Continued)

Substance Abuse Questions

Describe when and where you typically use substances ___Rare social drinking___

Describe any changes in your use patterns ___None___

Describe how your use has affected your family or friends (include their perceptions of your use)___

Reason(s) for use:

___ Addicted   ___ Build confidence   ___ Escape   ___ Self-medication

✓ Socialization   ___ Taste   ___ Other (specify)___

How do you believe your substance use affects your life? ___not___

Who or what has helped you in stopping or limiting your use? ___

Does (Has) someone in your family (present/past) have (had) a problem with drugs or alcohol? ✓ No ___ Yes (describe)___

Have you had withdrawal symptoms when trying to stop using drugs or alcohol? ✓ No ___ Yes (describe)___

Have you had adverse reactions or overdose to drugs or alcohol? (describe) ___NO___

Does your body temperature change when you drink? ✓ No ___ Yes (describe)___

Have drugs or alcohol created a problem for your job? ✓ No ___ Yes (describe)___

COUNSELING / PRIOR TREATMENT HISTORY

Information about **client** (past and present):

	No	Yes	When	Purpose ~~Where~~	Your reaction or overall experience
Counseling/Psychiatric treatment		✓	2000	Depression	It was helpful. Things got better.
		✓	age 13	Problems with father	Don't remember
Suicidal thoughts/attempts	✓				
Drug/Alcohol treatment	✓				
Hospitalizations	✓				
Involvement with self-help groups (e.g. AA, Al-Anon, NA, Overeaters Anonymous)	✓				

(continued)

FIGURE 3.1 (Continued)

Information about **family / significant others** (past and present):

	No	Yes	When	Where	Your reaction or overall experience
Counseling/Psychiatric treatment	✓				
Suicidal thoughts/attempts	✓				
Drug/alcohol treatment	✓				
Hospitalizations	✓				
Involvement with self-help groups (e.g. AA, Al-Anon, NA, Overeaters Anonymous)					

Please check behaviors and symptoms that occur to you more often than you would like them to take place:

__Aggression	__Dizziness	__Irritability	__Sleeping problems
__Alcohol dependence	__Drug dependence	__Judgment errors	__Speech problems
__Anger	__Eating disorder	__Loneliness	✓Suicidal thoughts
__Antisocial behavior	__Elevated mood	__Memory impairment	__Thoughts disorganized
__Anxiety	✓Fatigue	__Mood shifts	__Trembling
✓Avoiding people	__Gambling	__Panic attacks	✓Withdrawing
__Chest pain	__Hallucinations	__Phobias/fears	__Worrying
__Cyber addiction	__Heart palpitations	__Recurring thoughts	__Other (specify)
✓Depression	__High blood pressure	__Sexual addiction	_____
__Disorientation	__Hopelessness	__Sexual difficulties	_____
__Distractibility	__Impulsivity	__Sick often	_____

Briefly discuss how the above symptoms impair your ability to function effectively. I don't feel like seeing anybody or going to work. Too many bad things have happened to me. I want to get better.

Any additional information that would assist us in understanding your concerns or problems I feel abandoned by life.

What are your goals for therapy? Feel good about myself

Do you feel suicidal at this time? ✓No __Yes (explain)_____

FOR STAFF USE

Sigmund Z. Adler, PhD   5-3-05
Therapist's Signature/Credentials   Date

Physician's Comments Have reviewed intake material and agree with treatment considerations and diagnoses. Recommend med referral.

Physical Exam: ✓Required __Not Required

Carl J. Erikson, MD   5-10-05
Physician's Signature and Credentials   Date
Certifies case assignment, level of care and need for exam

FIGURE 3.2
Initial Intake Including Biophysical Assessment

Adult Initial Assessment

Client's Name _John Doe_   Date___5-17-05___

Starting Time__10:00___ Ending Time__11:30___   Duration__90 minutes__

Session Type ✓90801   __Other_____

A. BIOPSYCHOSOCIAL ASSESSMENT

1) Presenting Problem _Depressed mood, fatigue, social withdrawal,_
   lack of motivation

2) **Signs and Symptoms** (DSM based) . . . . **Resulting in Impairment(s)**

(Include current examples; for treatment planning)   (e.g. social, occupational, affective, cognitive, physical)

The client describes feeling depressed for the past 10 months. Since the
death of his wife, as evidenced by usual dysphoric mood, low motivation,
social withdrawal, decreased concentration, fatigue, and anhedonia. It
has resulted in affective, occupational, and social impairment, as
evidenced by missing 10 days of work in the past month, significantly
decreased production at work, avoiding friends and activities
previously enjoyed on a regular basis, and sitting home most of the time.

3) **History of presenting problem**

Events, precipitating factors or incidents leading to need for services _Spouse passed away_
10 months ago. Since then symptoms of depression have
increased.

Frequency/Duration/Severity/Cycling of symptoms _Depressed most of the time. Current_
episode is not cyclical. Previously treated for depression in 1993
after divorce.

Was there a clear time when Sx worsened? _Death of spouse_

Family mental health history _None Known_

FIGURE 3.2 (Continued)

4) CURRENT FAMILY AND SIGNIFICANT RELATIONSHIPS   See Personal History Form

No close family relation

Strengths/support_____

Stressors/problems _Ex-Spouse & children avoid him leading to shame_

Recent changes _2nd spouse died. Was in a functional relationship_

Changes desired _Desires to restore relationship with children and spend more time._

Comment on family circumstances _Feels abandoned by all family, no support_

5) CHILDHOOD / ADOLESCENT HISTORY   See Personal History Form

(Developmental milestones, past behavioral concerns, environment, abuse, school, social, mental health)

Normal developmental milestones. States that he was physically abused as a child. Brief counseling at age 13 dealing with issues with father. Average school grades. Describes his family as "dysfunctional." Parents divorced when he was teenager, stayed with mother.

6) SOCIAL RELATIONSHIPS   See Personal History Form

Currently avoids most people.

Strengths/support _One close friend_

Stressors/problems _Refusing invitations from friends. Doesn't feel like socializing._

Recent changes _Until depressed was much more active socially_

Changes desired _Increase time with friends_

7) CULTURAL / ETHNIC   See Personal History Form

No significant cultural/ethnic practices

Strengths/support_____N/A_

Stressors/problems_____N/A_

Beliefs /practices to incorporate into therapy _No_

8) SPIRITUAL / RELIGIOUS   See Personal History Form

strong fundament Christian beliefs

Strengths/support _Belief in God as source of strength_

Stressors/problems _Not involved in any activities_

Beliefs /practices to incorporate into therapy _Undecided_

Recent changes _No longer attending church activities_

Changes desired _undecided_

9) LEGAL   See Personal History Form

No criminal history. Minor traffic violation. Upcoming Child Support hearing.

Status/impact/stressors _Much stress over court meeting in 2 weeks._

FIGURE 3.2 (Continued)

10) EDUCATION   See Personal History Form

High school graduate - Average intelligence.

Strengths Would like to take public speaking course someday

Weaknesses None

11) EMPLOYMENT / VOCATIONAL   See Personal History Form

Has worked as laborer most of life. Jobs last 4-10 years

Strengths/support History of stable employment all of life.

Stressors/problems Missing approx. 10 days of work per month. Low production.

12) MILITARY   See Personal History Form

Army 4 years Honorable discharge.

Current impact None Known.

13) LEISURE / RECREATIONAL   See Personal History Form

None at present

Strengths/support History of regular involvement recreationally.

Recent changes Dropped almost all activities since spouse died.

Changes desired Wants to return to previous activities.

14) PHYSICAL HEALTH   See Personal History Form

No Known health problems. Has set up appt for physical and
med eval. No medications.

Physical factors affecting mental condition None Known

15) CHEMICAL USE HISTORY   See Personal History Form and Substance Abuse Addendum

Occasional social drinking. No increase since death of spouse.
No history of CD.

Patient's perception of problem None

16) COUNSELING / PRIOR TREATMENT HISTORY See Personal History Form: Client and Family

Previous diagnosis of "dysthymia" five years ago when receiving marital
counseling. Brief counseling as teenager. 6 months counseling for
depression in 1993. Counseling helpful.

Benefits of previous treatment Returned to premorbid functioning in 6 months.

Setbacks of previous treatment None Known

Page 3

(continued)

FIGURE 3.2 (Continued)

B. DIAGNOSTIC INTERVIEW

MOOD   (RULE IN AND RULE OUT SIGNS AND SYMPTOMS: VALIDATE WITH DSM)

Predominant mood during interview __*Depression*__

Current Concerns   (give examples of impairments (i), severity (s), frequency (f), duration (d))

Adjustment Disorder (w/in 3 months of Identified stressor, Sx persist < 6 months after stressor, marked distressed)
__Depressed   __Anxiety   __Mixed Anxiety & Depression   __Conduct   __Emotions & Conduct   __Unspecified
Specify disturbance: __Acute (<6 months) ✓Chronic (>6 months) __*Criteria not met*__

Impairment(s) _social _occupational/educational _affective _cognitive _other _____
Examples of impairment(s) _____

Major Depression (2 or more wks): ✓Usually depressed or ✓anhedonia. (4+ of following): ✓wght +/- 5%/month, ✓appetite⊕/-,
__sleep +/-, __psychomotor +/-, ✓fatigue, ✓worthlessness/guilt, ✓concentration, ✓death/suidal ideation.
Other; _crying spells,✓withdrawal, __add'l. sx _____

Impairment(s)✓social ✓occupational/educational ✓affective _cognitive _other _____
Examples of impairment(s) *Avoiding friends, missing work 10 days of past month*
Low production (previously "high producer")

Dysthymia (2 or more years): ✓depressed most of time. (2+ of following): ✓Low/high appetite or eating, __ In/hypersomnia, ✓low
energy/fatigue, ✓low self-esteem, ✓low concentration/decisions, ✓hopelessness. Other *Previous diagnosis of*
dysthymia. Endorses symptoms as occurring since teenager.
Impairment(s) _social _occupational/educational ✓affective _cognitive _other _____
Examples of impairment(s) *Feels sad most of the time*

Mania (3+): __Grandiosity, __low sleep, __talkative, __flight of ideas, __distractibility, __goals/agitation, __ excessive pleasure.
__*Denies*__

Impairment(s) _social _occupational/educational _affective _cognitive _other _____
Examples of impairment(s) _____

Panic Attacks (4+, Abrupt development of): __palpitations, __sweating, __trembling, __shortness of breath, __feeling of choking,
__chest pain, __nausea, __dizziness, __light-headed, __derealization, __fear of losing control, __fear of dying, __numbness, __chills /hot flashes
__*Denies*__

Impairment(s) _social _occupational/educational _affective _cognitive _other _____
Examples of impairment(s) _____

Anxiety (GAD: 3+, most of time, 6 months): __restlessness, __easily fatigued, __concentration, __irritability, __muscle tension, __sleep disturbance
__*Denies*__

Impairment(s) _social _occupational/educational _affective _cognitive _other _____
Examples of impairment(s) _____

Other Diagnostic Concerns or Behavioral Issues
(E.g., __Dissociation, __Eating, __Sleep, __Impulse control, __Thought disorders, __Anger, __Relationships, __Cognitive, __Phobias,
__Substance Abuse, __Medical conditions, __Somatization, __Phobias, __Sexual, __PTSD.etc.)
__*Denies each*__

Impairment(s) _social _occupational/educational _affective _cognitive _other _____
Examples of impairment(s) _____

USE ADDITIONAL PAPER AS NECESSARY

FIGURE 3.2 (Continued)

MENTAL STATUS	(Check appropriate level of Impairment: N/A or OK signifies no known impairment. Comment on significant areas of Impairment.)

APPEARANCE

	N/A or OK	Slight	Moderate	Severe
Unkempt, disheveled	O	●	O	O
Clothing; dirty, atypical	●	O	O	O
Odd phys.characteristics	●	O	O	O
Body odor	●	O	O	O
Appears unhealthy	●	O	O	O

POSTURE

	N/A or OK	Slight	Moderate	Severe
Slumped	O	O	●	O
Rigid, tense	●	O	O	O

BODY MOVEMENTS

	N/A or OK	Slight	Moderate	Severe
Accelerated, quick	●	O	O	O
Decreased, slowed	O	O	●	O
Restlessness, fidgety	●	O	O	O
Atypical, unusual	●	O	O	O

SPEECH

	N/A or OK	Slight	Moderate	Severe
Rapid	●	O	O	O
Slow	O	O	●	O
Loud	●	O	O	O
Soft	O	●	O	O
Mute	●	O	O	O
Atypical (e.g., slurring)	●	O	O	O

ATTITUDE

	N/A or OK	Slight	Moderate	Severe
Domineering, controlling	●	O	O	O
Submissive, dependent	O	O	●	O
Hostile, challenging	●	O	O	O
Guarded, suspicious	●	O	O	O
Uncooperative	●	O	O	O

AFFECT

	N/A or OK	Slight	Moderate	Severe
Inappropriate to thought	●	O	O	O
Increased lability	●	O	O	O
Blunted, dull, flat	O	●	O	O
Euphoria, elation	●	O	O	O
Anger, hostility	●	O	O	O
Depression, sadness	O	O	●	O
Anxiety	●	O	O	O
Irritability	●	O	O	O

PERCEPTION

	N/A or OK	Slight	Moderate	Severe
Illusions	●	O	O	O
Auditory hallucinations	●	O	O	O
Visual hallucinations	●	O	O	O
Other hallucinations	●	O	O	O

COGNITIVE

	N/A or OK	Slight	Moderate	Severe
Alertness	●	O	O	O
Attn. span, distractibility	O	●	O	O
Short-term memory	●	O	O	O
Long-term memory	●	O	O	O

JUDGMENT

	N/A or OK	Slight	Moderate	Severe
Decision making	●	O	O	O
Impulsivity	●	O	O	O

THOUGHT CONTENT

	N/A or OK	Slight	Moderate	Severe
Obsessions/compulsions	●	O	O	O
Phobic	●	O	O	O
Depersonalization	●	O	O	O
Suicidal ideation	O	●	O	O
Homicidal ideation	●	O	O	O
Delusions	●	O	O	O

Estimated level of intelligence __Average__

Orientation ✓Time ✓Place ✓Person **x 3**

Able to hold normal conversation? ✓Yes __No

Eye contact __Normal__

Level of Insight
__Complete denial   __Slight awareness
__Blames others   __Blames self
__Intellectual insight, but few changes likely
✓Emotional insight, understanding, change can occur

Patient's view of actions needed to change __increase__
__social & recreational activities__

Comments

__No evidence of thought disorder.__
__Appeared depressed. Cried a few__
__times during the interview. He__
__describes his depression as__
__similar to past episode which__
__was alleviated in about 6 months.__
__Good prognosis__

(continued)

FIGURE 3.2 (Continued)

C) DIAGNOSIS VALIDATION

DIAGNOSIS 1 _Major Depressive Disorder_   Code _296.31_

DSM Criteria

Depressed most of time. past 10 months, significant weight gain,
high appetite., often fatigued, feelings of worthlessness, decreased
concentration, suicidal ideations

Examples of impairment/dysfunction _Missing 10 days month at work_
Social: avoiding most people.   Affective: usually sad
Additional Validation (e.g. testing, previous records, self report) _No testing_

DIAGNOSIS 2 _Dysthymic Disorder_   Code _300.4_

DSM Criteria

Usually depressed most of life. History of poor appetite, low energy,
low self esteem, feelings of hopelessness

Examples of impairment/dysfunction _Feels "blue" most of the time since_
teenager
Additional Validation (e.g. testing, previous records, self report) _Previous diagnosis of_
dysthymia

DIAGNOSIS 3 _____   Code _____

DSM Criteria

_____
_____
_____

Examples of impairment/dysfunction _____
_____
Additional Validation (e.g. testing, previous records, self report) _____
_____

FIGURE 3.2 (Continued)

Integrated Summary

Clinical Assessment / Diagnostic Summary

(Evaluate, integrate and summarize the following information: Background, medical, social, presenting problem, signs & symptoms and impairments. Tie these in with the patient's strengths and needs. Integration of data is more important than specific details.)

The client describes feeling depressed for the past 10 months, since the death of his wife, as evidenced by usual dysphoric mood, low motivation, social withdrawal, decreased concentration, fatigue, and anhedonia. It has resulted in affective, occupational, and social impairment, as evidenced by missing 10 days of work in the past month, significantly decreased production at work, avoiding friends and activities previously enjoyed on a regular basis, and sitting home most of the time.

He has a history of being prone to depression when under significant stress. Previous counseling has been beneficial. Was given a diagnosis of Dysthymia in 1993. Some counseling as a child.

Some history of physical abuse as a child and marginal dysfunction in the family relationship. He has a previous diagnosis of Dysthymia. Strengths include spiritual beliefs, a premorbid functioning level of high work production and vocational consistency. He desires to return to previous functioning. Weaknesses are in his current level of motivation which is impairing several areas in his life. He describes his family is marginally supportive, at most. Prognosis is good due to his desire to improve, high insight, and previous successful psychotherapy.

	Diagnosis	Code
Axis I	Major Depressive Disorder	296.31
	Dysthymic Disorder	300.4
Axis II	No diagnosis	071.09
Axis III	Defer to Physician	
Axis IV	occupational problems, economic stress, relationship conflicts	
Axis V	Current GAF = 63	

Sigmund Z. Adler, PhD   5-17-05

Therapist's Signature and Credentials   Date

"a subjective manifestation of a pathological condition. Symptoms are reported by the affected individual rather than observed by the examiner" (p. 828).

The clinician elicits symptoms from the client, including descriptors such as onset, frequency, antecedents, intensity, and duration (OFAID procedure), plus notes the resulting impairments in an effort to both determine the appropriate diagnosis and demonstrate medical necessity for services. The presenting problem should be reflected in the treatment plan; however, this may not be possible when the client is in denial or noncompliant. Clinical noncompliance is especially difficult in cases of third-party reimbursement because this client is likely to deny that impairments exist; thus there may be no clear evidence of medical necessity. Chapter 7 discusses documentation for the noncompliant client.

Throughout this book we'll follow John Doe, a client with depression, through the course of therapy to illustrate the proper documentation process at each stage. Additional case examples will further illustrate correct and incorrect documentation techniques.

Presenting Problem and Signs

The first step in the diagnostic intake session is to determine the client's presenting problem and record signs and symptoms.

THERAPIST: What brings you here today?
JOHN DOE (Client): I've been feeling down lately.

Clarification

If the presenting problem is unclear, the therapist should seek clarification.

T: Tell me what you mean by "feeling down."
JD: I feel like no one cares about me; I'm sad, and I don't want to go to work anymore.

Onset

Next, the therapist determines the onset of the problem.

T: How long have you been feeling this way?
JD: I've been just fine all of my life, but for the past ten months I have had no motivation.

Antecedents

The therapist should also investigate whether a specific event (antecedent) occurred that brought on the presenting problem.

T: Did something happen last year?
JD: Yes, my wife died, and now I just can't do anything.

Specific Examples of Impairments

Once the presenting problem is determined, the therapist should find out how the problem is impairing the client's normal functioning.

T: How has this affected your performance at work?
JD: Over the past several months I keep missing more and more work. I'm now on probation at work and could lose my job if I don't improve. My production is the lowest in my department.
T: How many days of work have you missed this month?
JD: At least ten.
T: What were your reasons for missing work?
JD: I just didn't feel like getting up, I have no motivation . . . I have no energy, so I called in sick or made something up.
T: Is there anything you enjoy doing at this time?
JD: No, nothing is pleasurable.

Frequency

It is necessary at this point for the therapist to determine how frequently the problem occurs or impacts the client's functioning.

T: How often do you feel depressed?
JD: I'm depressed almost all of the time. Seldom a day goes by in which I'm not sad all day long. I just can't think straight or keep my mind on things.

Comparison to Premorbid Functioning

Finally, the therapist compares the client's current state to premorbid functioning to determine a baseline for treatment.

T: How were things at work for you before your wife died?
JD: It was hard, but I did as well as anyone else. I seldom missed any work, and I was up for a promotion because of seniority.

T: Describe your social life before your wife passed away.

JD: I was outgoing. I went out with friends at least twice a week and loved to play on sports teams at least one time every week.

T: What is currently happening in your life socially?

JD: I sit home alone every evening and weekend. I avoid people at work and cringe at the thought of having to be with people.

T: Are there any other areas in which your life has changed in the past ten months?

JD: No, that's about it.

The following example illustrates poor documentation of John Doe's signs and symptoms discussed in the diagnostic assessment interview:

> Client is feeling down. Missing work. Few activities. Wife died. Problems at work.

This statement summarizes the topics and current stressors discussed during the intake session but does not demonstrate medical necessity for treatment. Mental health concerns are implied but not documented. In this instance, the vagary of the documentation rather than the therapist's ability will ultimately jeopardize the client's chances of receiving mental health services when the therapist petitions for preauthorization for treatment. Even if the client receives services, the therapist might ultimately wind up repaying the insurance company the cost of service if audited.

A case manager or an auditor does not have access to a session transcript to review the many concerns brought up in the interview. In this case, in a short time period the therapist adequately solicits the information needed to validate medical necessity for services; however, due to poor documentation skills, there is no evidence of significant impairment in the client's functioning.

Do not blame the auditor or case manager for denying services for a needy client if the documentation does not clearly portray the medical necessity for services. Clients in need of mental health treatment are best served by a therapist who can both deliver quality mental health services and document the scope of services.

The next example provides better documentation for John Doe's problem but still does not clearly describe the medical necessity for treatment:

> Client claims to feel depressed since death of his spouse last year. He is not performing adequately at work and has no current friendships.

Although this example somewhat documents areas of impairment (affect, occupational, and social), it does not provide diagnostic information concordant with the interview narrative. For example, it is expected that a person would feel depressed after the death of a spouse as part of the normal grieving process; however, John Doe's level of depression is more severe than this documentation suggests. Stating that a person has no current friendships might hint at social concerns but in itself does not provide evidence for medically necessary treatment.

The following example illustrates the proper documentation of John Doe's signs and symptoms. It identifies stressors, time periods, symptoms, and impairments noted in the interview. It also provides baseline data for later assessments of the effects of treatment. Taken together, these signs and symptoms suggest that treatment is medically necessary to restore John Doe to normal functioning:

> The client describes feeling depressed most of the time (*frequency*) for the past 10 months (*onset*), since the death of his wife (*antecedents*), as evidenced by usual dysphoric mood, low motivation, social withdrawal, decreased concentration, fatigue and lack of pleasure (*DSM-IV-TR validation of symptoms*). It has resulted in affective, occupational, and social impairment (*impairments*) as evidenced by missing 10 days of work in the past month, significantly decreasing production at work, avoiding friends and activities previously enjoyed on a regular basis, and sitting home most of the time.

This portion of the diagnostic interview does not go so far into depth as to rule out specific disorders but instead focuses on signs and symptoms of the presenting problem. The presenting problem supplies baseline information that provides initial direction for the diagnostic interview. Further evidence of specific issues, personality disorders, and other concerns will be elicited later in the interview. As well, additional diagnostic information will continue to be formulated throughout therapy.

STEP TWO: History of Present Illness

The client's personal history statements provide valuable information regarding the client's past and present behaviors. It may be helpful in predicting future performance. Information such as strengths and stressors that tend to alleviate or increase problem

FIGURE 3.3

Domain Areas Required to be Investigated in Biopsychosocial Assessment

Family and Significant Relationships	Military
Childhood and Adolescent History	Leisure/Recreational
Social Relationships	Physical Health
Cultural/Ethnic	Chemical Use
Spiritual/Religious	Counseling/Prior Treatment
Legal	History
Employment/Educational	

areas are necessary in completing a treatment plan that is specifically designed for the client's needs. Previous mental health and physical health diagnoses help the therapist recognize behavior patterns that may be dysfunctional. Information may come from a variety of sources and draw from several domains in the client's life. Regulatory agencies, such as JCAHO, require that the assessment process address a number of areas (Figure 3.3).

In addition to recording this information, the therapist documents how these areas are impacting the client's current functioning. The information is directly integrated into the treatment plan and incorporated into therapy. Figure 3.4 describes the type of information that should be elicited and demonstrates its clinical significance.

The following dialogue between John Doe and his therapist demonstrates how to elicit specific client information related to the domain areas specified in Figure 3.3 to use in treatment planning. It defines measurable behaviors that both John Doe and the therapist view to be helpful in restoring and maintaining appropriate mental health. The therapist does not provide therapy at this point but, rather, identifies target information for future sessions and current diagnostic significance.

Family and Significant Relationships

T: Tell me about your family.

JD: Since my wife died. . . . my second wife. . . . I haven't been in contact with her family. I have two children from my first marriage, but they live with their mother.

T: How about your immediate family?

JD: They moved across the country a few years ago. They can't afford to visit me. The last time I saw them was at my wife's funeral. We've never been that close, though.

FIGURE 3.4
Type of Information Solicited for Biopsychosocial Domains and Its Clinical Significance

Solicited Information	Clinical Significance
Strengths/supports	Incorporate into treatment plan to most effectively integrate client's existing strengths and supports available from a wide range of areas.
Stressors/problems	Identify current problem areas that may be contributing to the client's mental health issues; also important diagnostically to justify an adjustment disorder.
Recent changes	Change in itself, whether viewed as positive or negative, often results in a stressful reaction. Note the client's reaction to changes and the permanence of the changes.
Changes desired	Document in the objectives section of the treatment plan and implement using various intervention techniques.
Specific beliefs or practices	Cultural, ethnic, and religious beliefs and practices should be identified prior to beginning treatment. Lack of knowledge in these areas is usually counterproductive, especially when counseling practices might contradict deep-rooted systems or beliefs.
Development —Past behavioral concerns —Past abuse —School issues —Social information —Mental health —Family dynamics	The clinical use of previous history is important because it may provide clues as to the etiology of current behaviors, responses, coping mechanisms, strengths, and disabilities. It helps the therapist to understand difficult developmental issues affecting current behaviors. Much of this information can be obtained from documents filled out by the client prior to the intake session.

T: Do you have any friends here?

JD: I see one of my high school friends about once every month or two.

T: When you need to talk to someone about personal issues, who is available or with whom do you feel comfortable?

JD: Certainly not my first wife. She has always poisoned our two children against me so much that they don't even want to visit me on weekends. My ex-wife digs it in that I'm depressed and not a good example for the children.

T: Do you have any relatives you can talk to?

JD: Sometimes I phone my brother in Detroit to complain about things, but he seems to side with my ex-wife. They used to date. I think they're still in touch.

T: What about your friend?

JD: Our relationship is mainly competitive . . . you know . . . like playing pool and shooting hoops. Lately, though, I've canceled our engagements. When we're together we want to have fun. If we talked about problems it would take away from the escape.

T: So are you saying that being with your friend helps on another level?

JD: What do you mean?

T: It sounds like being with him is a helpful escape from your problems.

JD: I never thought of it that way . . . yes.

T: Tell me more about how your children impact or affect your mood.

JD: I just feel lower and lower. I sit home and mope and feel so bad that I'm embarrassed to see the children. I used to take them at least two places every week. It's not happening. Nothing good is happening with my family. I have a dead wife, an ex-wife, and an ex-family.

T: It sounds like things used to be much better. What changes would you like to see in your relationships?

JD: If I could change anything it would be to have fun with my children.

T: How much time do you now spend with your children?

JD: About two hours a week when they want to see me.

T: How much time would you like to spend with them?

JD: At least ten hours a week, doing things we used to do. I have liberal visitation rights . . . at least on paper.

T: What about your relationships with other people in your life?

JD: I would like to spend more time with my best friend. Things always feel better when we go out and spend time together. It takes my mind off of things.

T: How often do you see him now?

JD: Not in the last three months.

T: How often would you like to see your friend?

JD: At least once or twice a month.

Childhood and Adolescent History

T: Tell me about your childhood.

JD: For the most part it was fairly uneventful. My parents got along about half the time. I had friends and did well in school. I never got in trouble with the law or in school.

T: Did you ever see a counselor or have any emotional or behavioral problems when you were a child or adolescent?

JD: Well, once when I was about thirteen I threatened suicide when my father punished me for something I didn't do.

T: Go on.

JD: My father always accused me of not being obedient and then beat me. He did this several times when I was younger. My mother eventually kicked him out of the house. After that our home life was tolerable.

T: You mentioned threatening suicide.

JD: I was so stressed out that I didn't feel I could go on any longer. School was getting to be too difficult, I hated my father, and my friends made fun of me because they often heard my parents fighting. I just wanted to give up. I really wouldn't have killed myself, but I didn't want to be around, either. My mother took me to a counselor, and after about two or three months I felt better.

T: How has handling change been for you at other times?

JD: Actually, I've never been good at changes. I usually get depressed and isolate myself. I don't like any challenges. I like feeling comfortable and secure.

T: How was your school and social life as a child?

JD: I always had friends. People treated me okay, especially after my father left. Things were then calmer at our house. I had average grades in school. I was okay.

Social Relationships

T: Tell me about your social life.

JD: What social life? I have none.

T: Are you presently involved in any activities or see any other people than those you mentioned?

JD: No, not really. I don't feel like it.

T: How long has it been since you did any socializing?

JD: Not since my wife died. Most of our friends were married. Now we have nothing in common.

T: Is there anything you miss about being with people or going out?

JD: I used to like just talking to people. I was a real people person. I could talk to anybody. But it's like I forgot how or have no motivation to do it.

T: How would you like things to be?

JD: I guess if things were better, I'd like to be involved in some sort of recreational activity but not now.

Cultural/Ethnic

T: Do you have any cultural or ethnic beliefs or practices which would be helpful for me to know or which would be helpful to the counseling processes?

JD: No, not really . . . I'm a White, middle-class, Anglo-Saxon Protestant.

Spiritual/Religious

T: Are there any spiritual or religious beliefs that would be helpful for me to know?

JD: Yes, I am a born-again Christian. I always pray before I make a major decision. I was raised with very strict rules of conduct and do not want any advice in counseling that would violate biblical principles.

T: Could you give me an example of what you mean?

JD: Sure, I don't believe in premarital sex; therefore, I hope you don't say I should seek sexual fulfillment in that manner. But at the same time, I believe that there is strength available from God if I put him first in my life and read positive passages from the Bible.

T: Tell me more about how the spiritual aspects of life can be positive for you.

JD: Although I haven't been to church since she died, I believe that Christians can help and support each other. I used to be very involved in church but stopped going when she died.

T: Do you think that this could be another avenue to help you at this time?

JD: I don't know if I'm ready yet.

T: What changes, if any, would you like to see in this area?

JD: Well, I used to feel more inner peace when I went to church. I don't want to talk about this now.

Legal

T: Are there any current legal concerns affecting you in any way?

JD: No, I've never been arrested for anything other than minor traffic violations.

T: Is there any court involvement at all at this time?

JD: Well, yes, I'm going through some child-support battles. We will go to court again in about two weeks.

T: How is this affecting you?

JD: Every day it annoys me. I can't afford the amount of support she is asking for. I feel like when I go to work my check is totally to pay for a house I no longer live in. So why should I even go to work? It's not fair at all. I'm still paying for funeral expenses. How can I have a life if all I do is pay money to my ex-wife to support children who don't even want to visit me?

T: It sounds like you are really frustrated about this.

JD: Yes . . . there is no room for me anymore. I can't do anything . . . it's like they own me, and the law is on their side.

Employment / Education

T: You said before that you have been missing a lot of work. Tell me more about it.

JD: I just have no motivation to go to work. Nothing is satisfying anymore. I used to be a top producer, but now it just doesn't matter because I have no reason to get ahead. The more I make the more my ex-wife gets and the more frustrated I become. Most of the time I'm just too down to feel like I'd be any good at work. What good could I do at work if I can't produce? I guess I'm just a loser. What else can I say?

T: What do you want it to be like at work?

JD: I wish that things were like the way they were before. I made good money . . . I was needed . . . I had goals . . . I never missed work. I really want to be that way again. That's why I'm here. I need a boost.

T: Are there any changes you would like to see educationally?

JD: I have always wanted to take a course in public speaking, but believe me, I'm in no mood right now to do that . . . maybe someday.

T: Someday?

JD: Yes, when I feel better about life.

Military

T: I see on your Personal Information Form that you were in the military. How was it for you?

JD: It was a learning experience. I did my time and survived. I didn't see any action. It was a job. It paid for my schooling. No problems.

Leisure / Recreational

T: What sort of things do you do for fun?

JD: Well, right now just about nothing, anymore.

T: Anymore?

JD: I used to be involved in plenty of activities.

T: Tell me about them.

JD: Okay. My second wife, the one who died, and I used to go to at least one sports event every two weeks, and we went to one cultural event every two weeks. The sports were for me, and the culture was for her. Actually, after a while we began to enjoy things together.

T: It sounds like you used to be pretty active in a number of areas.

JD: That's right . . . I used to be.

T: Tell me some more of the activities you used to like.

JD: Golfing, bowling, football games, basketball, antique stores, concerts, and going for walks.

T: That's quite a list. Do you miss some of them now?

JD: I do, but I always did them with her. About the only fun I have is with my best friend now and then.

Physical Health

T: How is your physical health?

JD: Oh, it's always been pretty good . . . lately I've felt fatigued, but I'm pretty healthy.

T: When was your last physical or visit to the doctor?

JD: About two years ago I had a physical for work. Everything was fine.

T: Do you have a history of any physical problems?

JD: No, I've always been in good health.

T: How about your family, such as your parents, siblings, or grandparents?

JD: Well, my father and grandmother had some thyroid problems, but I don't know too much about it. Overall, we're a pretty healthy family.

Chemical Use

T: Do you use alcohol or any other drugs?

JD: Yes, I drink socially on occasion, but it is not a problem.

T: How often is that?

JD: Oh, I might drink a few beers once every few months.

T: How does it affect you, or why do you drink?

JD: Just to fit in socially. I don't even enjoy the taste, especially.

T: When did you have your last drink?

JD: About six months ago. I had one glass of wine at an office party.

T: Have you ever had any problems with alcohol or any other drugs?

JD: No, I've never even been drunk. I've never tried any other street drugs.

T: Is there any chemical abuse history in your family?

JD: Not that I know of.

Counseling / Prior Treatment History

T: I noticed on your information form that you were in counseling about five years ago. Tell me about it.

JD: Well, I saw Dr. Bauste for individual therapy about five years ago for depression after my first wife and I were talking about a separation. It was similar to now. I just had no motivation to do anything, and I started missing work. Also, I already told you about some counseling as a teenager.

T: How did the therapy with Dr. Bauste turn out for you?

JD: We met every week for about six months. About half the time my wife attended the sessions. She suggested that I visit the psychiatrist for medications, but I was afraid to, so I didn't. Toward the end of counseling things seemed to get back to normal in our marriage, and I stopped missing work.

T: Was there anything in the counseling that was especially helpful?

JD: I don't remember the specifics, but Dr. Wilson often suggested things we could work on together to help the relationship. It seemed to work . . . at least for a while.

T: Do you remember if a diagnosis was given?

JD: I believe she said "Dysthymia" or something like that.

T: Later, we'll go over this and see how it relates to you today. It would be helpful if we could write to Dr. Wilson for your previous counseling records. Would that be all right?

JD: Sure.

T: Tell me about the other time you were in counseling.

JD: Like I mentioned before, I went to counseling at age thirteen because I had to please my father. You know, it made me appear as the sick person, instead of him.

T: Do you think it was helpful being there?

JD: No, not then, but counseling was okay when I went in 1993.

Interview information can be the most important data available to the clinician. Therefore the quality of the information and how it is used is crucial to the assessment and treatment plan process.

STEP THREE: Client Strengths and Limitations

Throughout the entire interview, client strengths and weaknesses are assessed in all areas. JCAHO requires that this information be incorporated into the treatment plan. The previous interview questions can help a therapist document client strengths and weaknesses so that they can be incorporated into counseling (Figure 3.5).

Although every client strength and weakness cannot be written directly in the treatment plan, the plan reflects these capabilities in order to provide more efficacious treatment. For example, if a client has good insight, the therapist might consider using insight-oriented therapy in treatment. On the other hand, if a client

FIGURE 3.5
Documenting John Doe's Strengths and Weaknesses

Strengths	Weaknesses
Recreational activities with best friend take his mind off problems	Little family contact
	His children avoid him
Motivated to increase time with others	Childhood relationship problems with father
History of having friendships	
Strengths in religious/spiritual beliefs	History of difficulty coping with change
Law abiding	Little/no social life at this time
History of stable work record	Stressed due to upcoming court visit (child support)
History of good physical health	
No history of chemical dependency	Missing much work lately
Successful counseling in past	Current low energy
Good insight	Low motivation

has severe cognitive deficits but responds well to specific, concrete behavioral intervention, behavior therapy could be more fitting. Clients with supportive social contacts would most likely respond well to incorporating this support into the treatment, whereas someone with a Social Phobia might panic if others were included immediately.

Information about client strengths and limitations may be solicited from a variety of sources including observations; questioning during the interview; prediagnostic questionnaires; collateral information, such as reports from other providers or family members; or psychological testing. Knowledge of the client's strengths and weaknesses, as with most clinical information, increases with time and rapport and may be incorporated into treatment throughout the course of therapy. Figure 3.6 lists categories similar to *DSM-IV-TR*'s examples of impairments and represents common strengths and limitations to consider during treatment planning.

SNAPs

In addition to collecting specific diagnostic information, a thorough assessment includes obtaining sufficient details about the client's **s**trengths, **n**eeds, **a**bilities, and **p**references (SNAPs; Wiger & Huntley, 2002). The SNAPs information may be collected from multiple sources (e.g., client statements during the interview, forms filled out by the client before or after the interview, collaterals, observations, previous records) and is incorporated into the clients' treatment to best suit their needs. Such information aids in viewing and understanding clients more in terms of being people, rather than as diagnoses.

Strengths

Strengths are discussed in the previous paragraph.

Needs

Client needs are specific areas of treatment of services that are current deficits in the client's life. Although the therapist cannot treat every client need, they can be addressed through actions such as referrals, handouts, additional services, homework assignments, and specific treatment plan objectives. Client needs could range from basic necessities, such as food, shelter, and clothing, to education to finding a physician to leaving an abusive relationship.

FIGURE 3.6
Examples of Areas of Client Strengths or Limitations That
May Be Incorporated into the Treatment Plan

Social

Accepts feedback	Helpful
Accepts responsibility for own behavior	Impulse control
Appropriately accesses support system	Listens to others
Articulate	Maintains appropriate boundaries
Assertive	Makes own decisions
Aware of impact on others	Organization membership(s)
Congruent	Outgoing
Dependable	Respectful
Empathic	Sense of humor
Establishes appropriate boundaries	Sensitive
Friendly	Sharing
Fun-loving	Supports others
Genuine	Tolerant of others
Good hygiene	Willing to please
Has long-term relationships	

Occupational/Educational

Abstract thinker	Good follower
Adapts to changes	Good leader
Articulate	Hard worker
Assertive	Independent
Attention span good	Learns fast
Aware of impact on others	Logical
Bright	Organized
Common sense good	Reads well
Concentration	Reliable
Concrete thinking	Stable employment
Cooperative	Team player
Creative	Uses lists
Dedicated	Willing to please
Dependable	Works hard
Goal focused	Writes well

Affective

Accepts feelings in self	Empathic
Accepts feelings in others	Expresses emotions
Aware of feelings	Integrates thinking and feeling
Aware of impact of feelings on behavior	Range of feelings available
Emotions appropriate	Tolerates emotional discomfort

FIGURE 3.6 (Continued)

Cognitive

Abstract thinker	Insight into own behavior
Attention/concentration	Insight into others' behaviors
Aware of how thoughts affect feelings	Intelligent
Aware of how thoughts affect behaviors	Logical
Clear imagery	Memory
Creative	Positive self-dialogue
Delays decision making	Reality testing intact
Flexibility in thinking	Reflects on own behavior

Physical

Eats well	Healthy
Endurance	Maintains normal weight
Exercises regularly	Solid sleep

Note: Provided by Danielle Jordan, PhD. MN School of Professional Psychology at Argosy University/Twin Cities.

Abilities

Client abilities can be a significant component in successful mental health treatment. The question, "What is the client able to do?" is addressed. If a therapist inappropriately suggests a behavior that the client is not able to do, no positive results will take place. For example, if attending a specific group seems likely to help the client but the client is not able to get on a bus or get a ride there, nothing would become of the strategy. Some therapists suggest that clients read certain books as bibliotherapy, but if they are not able to afford the books, nothing will be accomplished.

Preferences

Client preferences have historically been overlooked by some therapists. Treatment may involve a number of preferences in which the client is given a choice in areas such as type of therapy, frequency of visits, time of visits, use of collaterals, and treatment plan objects. Too many clients have terminated therapy prematurely because the entire therapeutic process was dictated by the therapist, and no choices were available.

The Psychological Report

Report writing is one of the most important skills a mental health professional can learn. The psychological report is typically the only mechanism of communicating a client's psychological, cognitive, personality, adaptive, and other types of functioning. A mediocre report reflects directly on the perceived clinical ability of the writer. A concise, insightful, information-filled report speaks highly about the clinician and will typically generate future referrals.

The psychological report (see example in Appendix A), also known as or is similar to an integrated summary, a psychological evaluation, a consultative examination, or a clinical assessment, provides a technically accurate yet concise overview of the client's psychological functioning. The psychological report integrates all aspects of the information collected during preinterview screening and the initial intake. Several different psychological report formats exist, but the specific order or outline of the presentation of information is not as important as the overall content and integration of material. Reports should be written to be easily understood by both mental health professionals and nonclinicians. Unclear reports result in loss of future referrals and, often, much postreport time spent answering questions that could have been covered in the report.

Different readers may focus on different aspects of the report depending on their level of understanding and reason for reading the report. Some readers focus on raw data and observations, whereas others prefer reading the diagnosis and recommendations. Overall, the report should be written so that the client can understand it; however, the report should also provide enough details to portray an accurate clinical picture. Using excessive technical jargon is unnecessary, especially because the report is meant to be summative. There are at least six sources for integrating information into the psychological report, including the following:

1. Clinical information collected by the clinician during the interview

2. Biographical information collected from preinterview screening such as information gathered in forms or telephone prescreening

3. Information from other professionals who have treated the client

4. Behavioral observations made during the initial interview

5. Test results (e.g., personality, cognitive, behavioral, adaptive functioning)

6. Information from collaterals such as significant others, teachers, bosses, friends, or family members

Effective writing skills are necessary to clearly integrate the several sources of information. In addition, reporting raw data from tests or observations is meaningless without integration and interpretation. Consider the difference between the following three statements:

1. "The client's MMPI-2 score indicated elevated scores in the 2, 4, and 7 scales."

2. "The client's MMPI-2 score suggested concerns with depression, anger, and anxiety. People with similar profiles tend to exhibit behavior cycles of acting out, guilt, and subsequent depression."

3. "The client's MMPI-2 score indicated elevated scores in the 2, 4, and 7 scales and suggested concerns with depression, anger, and anxiety. People with similar profiles tend to exhibit behavior cycles of acting out, guilt, and subsequent depression."

The first statement might be significant to someone trained in using the Minnesota Multiphasic Personality Inventory—2nd ed. (MMPI-2). The second statement is understandable to people not trained in clinical interpretation. Both types of information are found in statement three, which is intended to be understood by any reader; however, statements in this format tend to be lengthier than the others. If a report has only one intended type of readership (e.g., mental health professionals only), it would save time by not including simple language solely for the sake of explanation of clinical terms (as in statement one).

Factors influencing the report's format include its purpose (the referral question), the writer's theoretical orientation, the intended audience, and the writing style. The same writer will often write reports that look different depending on the purpose for which the report will be used. For example, if a report is primarily intended for the parent of a client to read, it will most likely be summative, rather than providing extensive test results or uninterpreted data. A report that is written for professionals may contain extensive clinical nomenclature and test scores. This text is not concerned about the particular format used to write the report; rather, it focuses on how to properly document information included in the report.

Psychological reports also vary in length. If a clinician includes all of the information gathered about a client, the report could easily reach 25 or more pages. Clinicians who provide little technical information and instead focus on integrating results could produce a report of only a few pages. This writer suggests providing adequate details pertaining to the referral question and summarizing other areas. For example, some clinicians administer a standard test battery to every client as a screening process. If the referral question is, "Does this person qualify for an anger management group?" it may not be important to extensively interpret intellectual tests. But in the case of a brain injury, the interpretation of these tests may be extremely important. It is the practice of this psychologist, when a referral for a psychological evaluation is received, to discuss with the referral source what types of information are desired in the report.

In the not-so-distant past, clinicians routinely administered a standard battery of tests to clients. However, due to payment authorization issues, the practice of administering a seemingly unlimited number of tests has declined. Often the clinician decides which specific tests and procedures to administer after sufficient rule-in/rule-out questions (described in Chapter 5) have been answered and a clearer clinical picture is presented. In actual clinical practice, it is becoming more common to have each intended test preapproved to secure preauthorization of payment.

Diagnostic and biopsychosocial information continues to be collected and revised throughout the course of therapy, and adjustments to the treatment plan are made as needed. Some clinicians prefer to wait a few weeks before filling out a biopsychosocial report until they have received adequate collateral information and have attained sufficient information in the sessions. Once the initial biopsychosocial assessment is complete, the next step in the initial intake is to conduct a mental status exam. Chapter 4 introduces several components that can be used to determine a client's current mental state.

HIGHLIGHTS
of Chapter 3

* The biopsychosocial assessment provides historical information from several areas of a client's life. Both strengths and weaknesses are incorporated into treatment planning.

* Biopsychosocial information may be gathered from several sources including questionnaires, clinical questioning, and collateral information.

* Although the purpose of the diagnostic interview is to gather information, it can be both informative and therapeutic by increasing client insight due to the nature of the questions and answers.

* The documentation of both signs and symptoms provides current information regarding mental health symptoms from the client's and therapist's perspective.

* The only clinical information available to a third-party auditor or case manager is that which is furnished by the therapist; therefore, inadequate documentation will result in denial of services.

* The best predictor of future behavior is past behavior.

* Three steps of conducting a biopsychosocial assessment include collecting information for (a) the presenting problem, (b) history, and (c) strengths and weaknesses.

* Assessing client strengths and weaknesses helps determine which types of interventions may be the most appropriate.

* The psychological report should be written in a level of technical language concordant with the intended reader(s).

QUESTIONS

1. The biopsychosocial assessment focuses on
    (a) background information.
    (b) current mental status.
    (c) clinical diagnosis.
    (d) future behaviors.

2. Signs are_____ and symptoms are _____.

    (a) endorsed by the client/observed by the clinician

    (b) observed by the clinician/endorsed by the client

    (c) physical/psychological

    (d) observable/implied

3. Which of the following best incorporates portions of the OFAID procedure?

    (a) The client has been depressed since his divorce.

    (b) The client is depressed almost all of the time.

    (c) The client is severely depressed.

    (d) All of these.

4. How are client strengths and weaknesses typically incorporated into a treatment plan?

    (a) They are specifically listed in the treatment plan.

    (b) They are incorporated into the treatment strategies.

    (c) Only weaknesses are incorporated because of the medical model.

    (d) Only strengths are incorporated due to a positive focus.

5. Which of the following is *not* part of the biopsychosocial assessment?

    (a) spiritual matters

    (b) drug and alcohol use

    (c) clinical observations

    (d) friendships

6. Written psychological reports should

    (a) be written in a concise, scientific, and technical manner.

    (b) primarily focus on the diagnosis.

    (c) be read only by professionals.

    (d) be written at a level concordant with the reader's level of understanding.

Answers: 1. a; 2. b; 3. d; 4. b; 5. c; 6. d

4

The Mental Status Exam

The mental status exam (MSE), an essential part of the diagnostic interview, is administered through both questioning and observations. Where the biopsychosocial assessment primarily focuses on history, the MSE's focal point is the client's current mental state. It includes making several observations about the client designed to clarify, validate, and compare clinical information that has been received. Mental status exam observation sometimes seems to contradict previous records because it represents the client's mental status "here and now," rather than previous behaviors. That is, a typically normal functioning client, during a time of stress, could exhibit significant concerns during the MSE and rather quickly return to normal functioning when the stressor has alleviated. Or, vice versa, a typically dysfunctional client could present in a normal manner at the time of the interview. Therefore, a psychological report that integrates historical and MSE information provides a wealth of clinical information.

The MSE was adapted from the physical examination that reviews major organ systems, while the MSE reviews major psychiatric functions. Mental status exam formats, such as the Mini Mental Exam (Folstein, Folstein, & McHugh, 1975), are widely used. However, most MSEs are conducted informally. In general, the greater degree of mental impairment, the more focus the MSE receives. That is, if a client's concerns are minor affective issues or behavioral problems, the MSE may not reveal any specific mental status issues other than current affective state. But clients presenting with severe psychotic, cognitive, behavioral, or affective concerns may readily reveal mental status concerns.

It is not common to administer a MSE to children; however, observations and parental statements tend to focus on similar information. Many clinicians do not ever formally conduct a MSE, but their clinical observations and notations serve the same purpose. This writer suggests incorporating a separate topic of "Mental Status Exam" in psychological reports because it assures the reader that the information in that section is a current mental status snapshot rather than historical information.

Whether conducted formally or informally, the MSE evaluates items such as the client's appearance, posture, speech, and judgment. It is not conducted in a specific time during the diagnostic interview but is administered throughout the intake session as observations are noted. Nevertheless, mental status observations are generally documented in a separate section of the psychological report.

Without conducting a MSE, there is an increased risk of misdiagnosis, especially for clients with poor insight, thought disorders, or who are in denial. For example, a client might deny being upset or agitated, but the clinician may observe several such behaviors during assessment. Simply considering the client's responses to questions the therapist has posed will not help the therapist reach a diagnosis in such cases. The observations and clinical interpretive skills employed in the MSE will aid in differential diagnosis and will provide the therapist with cues regarding how to proceed with the intake.

As noted, MSE's are available in a variety of formats, but they seek similar information. Frequently, the information gathered in the MSE is presented as a checklist of items the clinician observes and documents in the assessment. The areas most commonly reported in a MSE include the following:

- Appearance
- Activity level
- Speech/Language
- Attitude
- Affect/Mood
- Stream of consciousness
- Sensorium/Cognition

APPEARANCE

Descriptors of appearance should be objective and include aspects such as the client's neatness and cleanliness of dress, grooming, hygiene, body odor, and apparent health. An unusual appearance could signify a number of concerns. For example, loud, expensive, or bright clothing is not unusual during a manic episode or may suggest a Cluster B Personality Disorder.

Inappropriate clothing *might* represent cognitive concerns or confusion of thought. Impeccable dressing, or a client who constantly straightens an article of clothing, *might* indicate obsessive-compulsive concerns. Depression, substance abuse, a thought disorder, or dementia *might* be depicted in clothing that is noticeably soiled, wrinkled, or foul in odor. However, a client's appearance alone should not be the basis of a diagnosis. The client's subculture, background, socioeconomic status, and current life situation must be taken into account before passing judgment. Never base a diagnosis solely on one type of observation. The liberty of individual differences must always be factored in before assigning a label to someone who happens to be different. Those involved in conducting psychological interviews cannot allow their world view to influence their observations of clients. Open-mindedness and specific training in diversity are crucial for mental health professionals. Consider a therapist's observations about the appearance of a client:

> Grant B. appeared at the interview wearing worn jeans and several layers of soiled clothing. He was 6 feet tall, weighed 120 lbs., and seemed to be poorly nourished. He appeared to be at least 15 to 20 years older than his chronological age of 48, as evidenced by a slumped posture, yellowed teeth, a rosy complexion, and disheveled hair. He appeared to be in below average health. There was a strong smell of alcohol on his clothing.

The information provided in the preceding paragraph is written in a fairly objective manner and makes no judgments; however, it could easily lead to premature conclusions. More information is needed regarding the context of the client's current situation. Consider how your evaluation (professionally and personally) of the client in the preceding narrative might change if the description was preceded by any of the following statements:

1. The client is applying for a job as a salesperson.
2. The client, a civil engineer, sustained a head injury from an assault when he was robbed of his possessions and clothing. Apparently, he was found and taken care of in an abandoned building by unknown persons.

3. The client was diagnosed with cancer 6 months ago.

4. This is the client's tenth time in chemical dependency (CD) treatment.

5. Three months ago, on the way to a "Helping Humanity" volunteer weekend, the client was backing up his car and accidentally ran over a child.

A report that integrates both MSE and background information clearly provides the reader with sufficient information to understand the client's condition and needs.

The client's posture may also indicate a variety of nonverbal attitudes, Pain Disorders, or levels of affect (e.g., slumped—signifying depression; leaning forward—signifying interest; erect—signifying anxiety or other concerns). Changes in the client's body position during the interview might signal pain, anxiety, or feelings of discomfort. It is not helpful to make premature judgments, but, rather, it is best to make ongoing hypotheses that may be ruled in and ruled out as more information is received.

Other information that can be gleaned from observing a client's appearance includes a description of whether the client's appearance matches his or her chronological age, facial expressions, level of eye contact, or any other unusual physical characteristics that could indicate psychological or physical dysfunction. It is not necessary to list every possible observation; rather, the clinician should report only those that may be clinically significant or affect the validity of the interview. Consider the observations in the context of the client's cultural background.

When the client's appearance appears to be normal, do not assume that the reader is aware of this information, but, rather, make statements such as, "The client appeared at the interview looking his chronological age. His posture, health, grooming, and hygiene appeared to be within normal limits."

Some of the possible observations (other than normal) of a client's appearance appear in Table 4.1.

ACTIVITY LEVEL

Activity level, body movements, and motor behaviors may reflect a wide range of psychological concerns. The clinician should report any unusual movements; otherwise, the report should indicate that the client did not exhibit abnormal body movement behaviors. Nu-

TABLE 4.1
Possible Observations of a Client's Appearance

Topic	Examples of observations	Narrative examples: "The client('s) . . .
Age	Younger/Older	. . . appears to be at least 10 years older than her chronological age."
Posture	Erect/Slumped/Shifting	. . . exhibited a slumped posture during the entire interview."
Grooming	Poor/Neat	. . . was groomed very poorly, as evidenced by . . . (give examples of the grooming)."
Hair	Clean/Dirty/Disheveled	. . . hair was uncombed, oily, and disheveled."
Nails	Clean/Dirty/Bitten/Long/ Neatly trimmed	. . . nails were very short, dirty, and appeared to be bitten."
Odor	Strong body odor/Smell of alcohol	. . . body odor was very strong, suggesting poor hygiene." (Note: consider cultural factors before making such statements.)
Health	Good/Poor	. . . appeared to be in good health." (Note: Do not make a medical-like diagnosis of good health. Simply make an observation of the appearance.)
Weight	Under/Over	. . . was morbidly obese, weighing 380 lbs."

merous clinical terms are available to describe various body movement behaviors; however, it is best to describe them in layman's terms. This makes reports more readily understandable yet preserves clinical integrity.

Some clinicians choose to incorporate technical terms in the report or describe behaviors in simpler terms, depending on the intended reader. Table 4.2 demonstrates the difference between clinical terminology and everyday language. Although the same message is being portrayed, the level of understanding is more widespread using everyday language.

Normal activity level might be described with statements such as, "No concerns were noted in the client's activity level. There were no unusual gestures or mannerisms. His activity level was within normal limits. He was not limp, rigid, lethargic, combative, or hy-

TABLE 4.2

Clinical Observations and Everyday Language Definitions of Observable Body Movements

Clinical Terminology	Everyday Language
Akathisia	The client reports feeling restlessness in legs since the onset of neuroleptics.
Akinesia	Few movements were noticed in areas such as arm movement when walking and eye blinking.
Athetoid movements	Slow, involuntary, snakelike movements were observed in the client's arms.
Choreiform movements	Quick, jerky, involuntary movements were noticed in the client's limbs.
Dystonia	The client's head remained twisted for several minutes, during which time the client's tongue remained stuck out.
Hypokinesia	Very few body movements were noticed such as the client's arms rarely moved when the client walked.
Masked facies	There was no facial expression.
Psychomotor agitation	The client had difficulties sitting still and appeared restless and tense.
Psychomotor retardation	Body movements and speech patterns were slow.
Waxy flexibility	Client's body position, in which arms were extended upward, remained unchanged despite all attempts to change it by staff.

peractive. He did not appear to be preoccupied or easily distracted. He sat still the entire time. He appeared to be relaxed and alert. Accessory movements were within normal limits."

It is not likely that every behavior listed in following observations would be listed in every report, but those that are clinically significant warrant mention. Some of the possible observations of a client's activity level are shown in Table 4.3.

SPEECH / LANGUAGE

Observing a client's speech provides important mental status and diagnostic information. Speech aphasia describes problems with grammar, word usage, and sentence structure. Unusual speech patterns may indicate affective, neurological, psychotic, physical, or cognitive dysfunction. Clinicians must be careful not to pass judgment based on speech patterns alone but, rather, use such informa-

TABLE 4.3
Possible Observations of a Client's Activity Level

Topic	Examples of observations	Narrative examples: "The client('s) . . .
Gestures/ Mannerisms	Unusual	. . . frequently blinked his eyes and clenched her fists."
Alertness	Low/High	. . . level of alertness was poor and needed several prompts to answer questions."
Kinetic	Hyperactive/Hypoactive	. . . was quite hyperactive throughout the session, frequently getting out of her chair."
Vigilance	Hypervigilant/Hypovigilant	. . . was extremely hypervigilant, frequently scanning the room and looking out the window."
Gait	Steady/Unsteady/Shuffled	. . . walked with an unsteady gait."
Eye contact	Poor/Excessive	. . . made little or no eye contact during the entire interview."
Relaxed	(Level of)	. . . appeared to be very relaxed."
Lethargic	(Level of)	. . . was quite lethargic."
Limp/Rigid	(Level of)	. . . movements and posture were rigid."
Distracted	(Level of)	. . . was easily and frequently distracted."
Preoccupied	(Level of)	. . . appeared to be preoccupied."
Accessory movements	(Decreased/Increased)	. . . exhibited decreased accessory movements."

tion as a piece of the puzzle to be integrated and concordant with other observations.

It can be difficult to differentiate between speech problems resulting from organic versus psychiatric etiology. Although symptoms tend to overlap, organic speech problems tend to be progressive, unless they follow a traumatic event such as a stroke. Psychiatric speech problems, on the other hand, tend to coincide with psychiatric episodes.

Although no clear standards are defined, the MSE should report any departures from what is considered functional. Because such information is based on opinion, observed examples should be provided. If no abnormal speech behaviors are evident, the therapist should note this as well. For example, the therapist might

TABLE 4.4
Possible Observations of a Client's Speech/Language

Topic	Examples of observations	Narrative examples: "The client('s) . . .
Vocabulary	Limited/Unusual/Superior	. . . vocabulary was significantly below average, concordant with intellectual functioning."
Details	Few/Excessive	. . . provided few details and often evaded a number of questions asked of her."
Pronunciations	Poor/Succinct	. . . pronunciations were poor, which is concordant with a history of speech therapy."
Sentence structure	Brief/Rambled/Unusual	. . . sentence structure was unusual in that every response was in the future tense."
Volume	Soft/Loud/Varied	. . . volume was very loud in the beginning of the interview but decreased significantly during the MSE."
Pace	Slow/Fast	. . . pace was quite rapid, concordant with his history of mania."
Neologisms	Unusual	"Several neologisms, such as _____ were noted, concordant with her history of Schizophrenia, Disorganized Type."
Repetitions	Excessive	. . . often repeated phrases such as _____, suggesting a possible thought disorder and/or obsessiveness."
Reaction time	Delayed/Immediate	. . . oftentimes responded to questions before the question was finished."
Pitch	High/Low	. . . voice was at an extremely high pitch."
Volume	Soft/Loud	. . . voice was very soft, and several responses had to be repeated."
Slurred	(Degree of)	. . . speech was slurred, which was concordant with stroke symptoms."
Tone	(Monotonous/Expressive)	. . . tone of speech was monotonous, suggestive of a depressed mood."
Stuttered	(Degree of)	. . . speech was stuttered only when discussing previous abuse."

TABLE 4.4

Topic	Examples of observations	Narrative examples: "The client('s) . . .
Mumbled	(Degree of)	. . . speech was severely mumbled to a degree in which it was barely understandable."
Echolalia	(Degree of)	. . . speech suggested echolalia, which is concordant with her previous diagnosis."
% Understood	(Estimate of %)	. . . speech was approximately 90% understandable."

record, "The patient expressed a normal range of vocabulary, volume, reaction time, details, pace, pitch, articulation, and spontaneity," or "No speech concerns were noted."

When abnormal speech patterns do exist, further observations, such as whether speech is pressured, hesitant, monotonous, slurred, stuttered, cluttered, mumbled, and whether repetitions, neologisms, difficulties with word finding, or echolalia are present, should be reported. In such cases, the therapist should document specific examples and incorporate them into the diagnostic summary.

Language observations go beyond the specific areas of speech. Therapists should evaluate and record the client's level of comprehension throughout the interview. Therapists also should document the client's ability to understand simple to complex requests or points of conversation. Some of the possible observations (other than normal) of a client's speech are shown in Table 4.4.

ATTITUDE TOWARD EXAMINER

The client's attitude toward the examiner is important in assessing areas such as relationship to authority, social behaviors in new situations, prognosis of treatment, and accuracy of information. In addition, Personality Disorder variables are often reflected in the client's attitude. Assessment is possible across several dimensions that should be considered on a continuum and include aspects such as level of interest, cooperation, frankness, defiance, evasiveness, defensiveness, guardedness, manipulation, hostility, hesitance, ability as historian, and sense of humor.

In the case of a cooperative client, a statement such as, "The client was cooperative, friendly, provided adequate historical information, and did not appear to be guarded or defensive," portrays a reasonable picture. When the client is not cooperative, the clinician should document abnormal behavior. For example, a clinician might write:

> Katie W. entered the office yelling at the receptionist, "All psychologists should be locked up." During the interview, she refused to answer over half of the questions, stating that they are no one's business. She made little eye contact and sat facing away. At one point she stated that she had not consumed alcohol in over six months; however, there appeared to be a strong odor of alcohol on her breath and clothing, noticed by three staff members and this therapist.

Therapists should integrate the purpose of the interview when making attitudinal observations. For behavioral disorders, clinicians should note observations relating to symptoms of the presenting problem. Some children (and adults) will behave differently in the waiting room than in the presence of the interviewer, so it is important to include observations of the client's behavior during the interview, as well as before and after the session, when possible. For example, children with Conduct Disorder may behave well during the interview but punch their parents or steal a magazine on the way out of the office. Likewise, children with Attention Deficit/ Hyperactivity Disorder (ADHD) may show no signs or symptoms of inattention or hyperactivity during the interview, but school records may indicate strong concerns. The *DSM-IV-TR* (APA, 2000) states that even though few or no symptoms may be observed in the clinician's office, a disorder may still be present.

In cases in which clinicians do not directly observe signs of a disorder, it is important to gather more information than usual from collaterals, such as family members or teachers. Generally, a provisional diagnosis and accompanying statements, such as "as per history" or "as per parent, but not observed during the interview," are used (e.g., 314.01 ADHD, Provisional, as per history [parents' comments, school records, psychiatrist's report], not observed during the interview).

Some of the possible observations (other than normal) of a client's attitude level are shown in Table 4.5.

An example of describing all areas of the client's attitude

TABLE 4.5
Possible Observations of a Client's Attitude toward the Examiner

Topic	Narrative examples: "The client('s) . . .
Attentiveness	. . . paid little attention to this examiner."
Cooperation	. . . was extremely uncooperative, refusing to answer most questions."
Friendliness	. . . was initially friendly, but when asked questions about his history of violence, he became quite irritable."
Manipulative	. . . was often manipulative by overly complimenting this examiner."
Matter of fact	. . . was not spontaneous and did not supply information other than that which was directly asked of her. She spoke in a matter-of-fact manner."
Humorous	. . . adequate sense of humor when describing daily activities."

toward the examiner is as follows: "He was cooperative and attentive and seemed interested in the interview. He appeared to be an adequate historian. He did not appear to be defiant, guarded, defensive, evasive, hostile, or manipulative."

AFFECT AND MOOD

Although often used interchangeably, affect and mood reflect the emotional state of the client from different perspectives. *Affect* refers to the clinician's observations of the client's emotional state, whereas *mood* represents the client's endorsement of symptoms. Affect and mood are usually congruent, but in cases of denial, defensiveness, or confusion, the clinician's observations may differ from the client's statements.

Affective observations include behavioral notations of the client's temperament during the examination. The following descriptors are often used in describing various aspects of affect.

Range of Affect

The affective range is on a continuum and is depicted from flat to normal. *Flat affect* is the total lack of affective responses. *Blunted affect* is characterized as a severely reduced level of affect. *Restricted affect* is a level noticeably below normal. *Normal affect* indicates that a typical and expected amount of affect was observed.

Appropriateness of Affect

The appropriateness of affect is the correspondence or correlation between the client's thoughts and speech versus the observed level of affect. For example, it would be unusual for a client to describe the recent traumatic loss of a loved one while giggling. Although appropriateness is often inconsistent in cases such as guardedness or denial, it may also indicate psychopathology.

Intensity of Affect

Affective intensity is characterized as the strength of emotional responses. For example, a person who sobs intensely with extreme emotional expression is described as having *strong intensity*, whereas someone who expresses little affect would be described as displaying *mild intensity*.

Mobility of Affect

Mobility of affect refers to the time span between changes in emotional expression. For example, *decreased mobility* (also referred to as *constricted mobility*) could refer to someone who does not show normal and expected changes in affect as topics of conversation change. *Increased mobility* or *lability* is exhibited by abrupt changes in emotional states, such as going from laughing to crying to anger in an unusually short time period.

Other descriptors of affect include psychomotor behaviors, level of anxiety, irritability, and anger expression. For example, if a client appears to be anxious but denies such concerns, the report might state:

> Steve M. often fidgeted with his fingers and bit his fingernails. On four occasions, he appeared perplexed and stuttered slightly. He often checked his watch, stating that he must get home before the rush hour or something bad might happen. But when asked if he describes himself as nervous, anxious, or worried, he adamantly denied any such concerns.

Mood

Mood is assessed by asking the client about his or her typical and current emotional state. This information is crucial diagnostically and is essential for the rule-in/rule-out process that will be covered in Chapter 5. Scores of human moods exist; however, most clinicians thoroughly assess emotional symptoms related to the *DSM-IV-TR* diagnoses. That is, although moods such as joy, surprise, and elation may be prevalent, they are typically not symptomatic of psychopathology, unless they are in excess or debilitating.

STREAM OF CONSCIOUSNESS

Stream of consciousness, also called *flow of thought,* is determined by observing speech patterns, which are presumed to indicate thought processes. Table 4.6 highlights relevant observations that can be made about a client's speech.

Flight of Ideas

An excessive number of ideas and rapid change in idea content denote a *flight of ideas.* The content of one idea has a relationship with the next or an idea may last for less than one sentence:

> We went to the store in the van. Traveling is just great. I love visiting the mountains, especially in the summertime. Oh, yes, the weather is great.

Associations

Loose associations refer to unrelated ideas that occur in the same sentence or within a few sentences. The words are coherent, but the content is not related and does not follow a logical sequence. Other types of associations (e.g., clang, derailment, tangentiality, and several others) also exist. Therapists should record specific examples in the psychological report. Other observations include excessive rambling, coherency of speech, logical speech, neologisms, cause and effect, and relevance of speech. These observations are rare and can indicate severe psychopathology.

> Why is whatever might be kind to others. You might think and do why not cobetize the plemil.

TABLE 4.6
Typical Speech Observations

Quality and Descriptions of Speech	Content of Speech
Vocabulary	Flight of ideas
Details	Loose associations
Articulation	Clang associations
Phraseology	Derailment
Volume	Tangential speech
Pace	Neologisms
Reaction time	Thought content
Pitch	Logical
Coherency	Cause/Effect
Repetitions	Relevance
Hesitancy	Hallucinations
Pressured	
Monotonous	
Slurred	
Mumbled	
Echolalia	
Rambling	
Word finding difficulties	
Mute	
Vocal tics	

Thought Content

Thought content refers to intrusive thoughts, unusual thoughts, destructive thoughts, or false beliefs that may preoccupy the client. Common preoccupations include obsessions, compulsions, phobias, or homicidal, suicidal, or antisocial thoughts. Thought disturbances, such as delusions of grandeur, persecution, or somatic concerns, may also be observed and recorded. Clinicians should also document ideas of reference such as thought broadcasting, bizarre ideations, and unusual content.

Terra B. states that she is constantly being watched by "agents of evil from another dimension." She further states that she has seen them in the television, and they are trying to recruit and possess her. She believes that if she "gives in" she will lose her soul.

Hallucinations

Hallucinations may be distortions of any of the five senses (optic, auditory, olfactory, tactile, or gustatory). Before noting such observations, the clinician should make certain that the client understands the context behind such questioning and that cultural and spiritual issues are considered. For example, if a highly religious person is asked, "Do you ever hear voices that no one else hears?" an affirmative answer does not necessarily imply a thought disorder. Instead, it could reflect a religious experience or a transient symptom of a severe affective disorder.

No matter what kinds of hallucinations are reported, it is important to clearly document the degree of the disturbance. Simply stating that hallucinations exist does not present a clear clinical picture. Similar to other signs and symptoms, it is important to document the onset, frequency, antecedents, intensity, duration, and resulting impairments of the hallucinations. Other notations of clinical significance related to hallucinations include depersonalization, derealization, déjà vu, overvalued ideas, and illusions, all of which suggest issues of perception.

SENSORIUM / COGNITION

This section of the MSE elicits information regarding the client's orientation, concentration, attention span, memory, and ability to hold a normal conversation.

Orientation × Three

This refers to the client's knowledge of the current time, place, and person. The therapist typically asks the client to state the time of day, date, year, and season; the name of the clinic and the city where the interview is taking place; and the client's name and the names of other important people in the client's life. Disorientation indicates cognitive dysfunction that could stem from a number of etiologies.

Attention and Concentration

Attention is the ability to focus on a given task, whereas concentration is the ability to sustain attention over a period of time. The MSE measures attention and concentration by recording the client's ability to perform various mental tasks. Examples of common attention and concentration tasks in the MSE include the following:

- Serial threes beginning with 1
- Serial sevens backward from 100
- Mathematical calculations
- Verbal tasks backward
- Repeating digits

Serial Threes

Clients are asked to count to 40 by threes beginning with 1 (e.g., 1, 4, 7, 10). The common margin of error is 0 to 2 mistakes, with an average of 2 to 3 seconds between digits. It is important to record the number of errors as well as the time that elapses between digits; the client's level of persistence, anxiety and frustration; and any strategies the client uses to perform the calculations in the report.

Serial Sevens from 100 Backward

This task is more difficult than serial threes. The normal margin of error is 0 to 2 mistakes, with an average of 3 to 6 seconds between digits. For this test, the client is asked to count backward from 100 by sevens. The clinician should make similar observations as the ones suggested for serial threes.

Mathematical Calculations

Depending on the client's level of education, the clinician can present mathematical calculations that are typically beyond rote memory. For example, adult clients might be asked to solve problems such as 65 divided by 5 and 12 multiplied by 6. Much simpler problems, such as asking a first grader to add 3 plus 4, are given to children.

Verbal Tasks Backward

Most adults are able to spell words such as *world* or *earth* forward, but during times of experiencing difficulty with concentration, errors are common when spelling words backward. Be sure to evaluate or estimate the client's intellectual level and any learning disabilities prior to making conclusions in such tasks. It is best to ask the client to first spell the words forward before attempting to spell them backward. If the client is not able to spell the word forward, choose a simpler word or select a new task. Other tasks include operations such as saying the months of the year backward or tasks that are not a challenge when recalled forward but are not typically performed backward.

Repeating Digits

The average adult is able to repeat 5 to 7 digits forward and 4 to 6 digits backward. The Wechsler intelligence test manuals provide child and adult norms for Digit Span. To administer the test, the therapist repeats an increasing number of digits, spaced one second apart and beginning with two digits forward, to the patient. The patient then repeats the digits back to the therapist in the same order. After a limit has been reached, the patient is asked to repeat another set of digits backward.

JUDGMENT

Judgment is assessed by asking the client direct questions about hypothetical situations in which choices of judgment must be made. Questions from the Wechsler Comprehension subtests are commonly used. Clinicians should bear in mind that although many clients are aware of what should be done in a particular situation, in real life they seldom take the best course of action. In this case, obtaining an accurate history of the client's behaviors will better support the clinician's determination of the client's judgment.

It is common to ask hypothetical questions such as, "What would you do if you were the first one in a theater to see smoke and fire coming from under one of the exit doors?" Observations include the quality of the answer and whether the answer is unusual. For example, if the client answers, "I'd yell fire," it is not an unusual response, but it may indicate lack of planning or impulsivity. An answer of, "I'd just leave," begs the question, "What about the other people?" Some clients will respond, "I would warn them as I left," whereas others would respond, "That's their problem." The query, in this case, provides valuable clinical information.

INSIGHT

A client's level of insight is important in assessing treatment prognosis. Lower levels of client insight generally indicate that the client will be less aware of psychological problems. Many therapists use more behavioral counseling methods for clients with poor insight and more cognitive methods for higher levels of insight. Levels of insight may vary from session to session or depend on the problem being addressed and include the following:

1. Complete denial
2. Slight awareness
3. Awareness, but blames others
4. Intellectual insight, but few changes likely
5. Emotional insight and understanding that changes can occur

Figure 3.2 (on pages 41–47) includes a mental status checklist on which the therapist documents various mental status dimensions. Some of the information is asked directly of the client, whereas other information is observed.

The biopsychosocial assessment, MSE, and other data collected from phone screens, presession questionnaires, and so on can be reviewed and integrated to assist the clinician in validating the diagnosis and demonstrating medical necessity for treatment. Chapter 5 explains the validation process.

HIGHLIGHTS
of Chapter 4

★ The MSE provides an index of the client's current mental condition. It is like a snapshot of the moment rather than being historical in nature.

★ The MSE is based on both behavioral, physical, and affective observations of the client and specific client statements.

* Mental status exam observations may vary from one session to the next, based on current mental status.

* Several specific MSE procedures are commonly employed to provide consistency and standardization.

* Observed speech, attitude, cognition, and affective observations are major components of the MSE.

* Thought content is generally assessed by the client's speech and language.

* The client's attitude and level of insight may be indicators of prognosis in therapy.

QUESTIONS

1. The *mental status exam* is intended to provide a(n)
   (a) summary of the client's past mental health history.
   (b) description of the reasons the client has come to therapy.
   (c) current picture of the client's current mental state.
   (d) overview of the client's past and present mental state.

2. Which of the following statements best represents a description of a client's affect?
   (a) "The client states that she is depressed, anxious, and irritable."
   (b) "The client states that she has previous diagnoses of depression and anxiety."
   (c) "The client appears to be depressed, anxious, and irritable."
   (d) Each of the above demonstrate a client's affect.

3. In a mental status exam, the client's *stream of consciousness* is evaluated by the client's
   (a) speech.
   (b) history.
   (c) affect.
   (d) IQ.

4. The client's mental status is evaluated
   (a) only during the mental status examine in the initial interview.
   (b) throughout treatment.
   (c) only when revising a treatment plan.
   (d) historically, every fourth session.

5. A client presents with slurred speech. This provides evidence of
   (a) alcoholism.
   (b) brain damage.
   (c) a Communication Disorder.
   (d) Need more information.

Answers: 1. c; 2. a; 3. a; 4. b; 5. d

5

Formulating and Validating a Diagnosis

Among the several purposes of the diagnostic interview is the need to document the medical necessity for services and solicit information to produce an accurate and effective treatment plan. Although it is not structured to be a counseling session, the manner in which information is solicited tends to be therapeutic for the client. If the therapist has a clear understanding of the *DSM-IV-TR* and psychopathology and shows empathy for the client's situation, the result will often aid client insight.

The *DSM-IV-TR* (APA, 2000) states, "In the *DSM-IV-TR*, each of the mental disorders is conceptualized as a clinically significant behavioral or psychological syndrome or pattern that occurs in an individual and that is associated with present distress (e.g., a painful symptom) or disability (i.e., impairment in one or more important areas of functioning) or with significantly increased risk of suffering death, pain, disability, or an important loss of freedom" (p. xxxi). It further explains that the syndrome must not be based on an expected behavior or culturally sanctioned behavior or a response to an event that would lead to an expected emotional reaction. The documentation process continuously monitors impairments and progress to justify the medical necessity of services.

Each *DSM-IV-TR* disorder is characterized by various diagnostic criteria such as symptoms, time frames, and impairments. Many disorders list a specific number of selected symptoms that must be present to justify the diagnosis. Symptom endorsement is necessary but not sufficient to make a diagnosis. Mental health diagnoses are not to be given in a cookbook-like fashion. That is, the process of formulating a diagnosis is not simply a matter of word processing in which a client endorses enough symptoms that the best fitting diagnosis is given. Questionnaires that base a diagnosis solely on endorsed symptoms clearly do not match the *DSM-IV-TR* criteria, because there are several other factors to consider when formulating a diagnosis.

The *DSM-IV-TR* cautions that the diagnostic criteria are guidelines meant to enhance communication among clinicians. The accuracy of *DSM-IV-TR* diagnoses is an ongoing work. Each revision since the first *DSM-IV-TR* has added specificity and has attempted to be a result of corroboration between mental health professionals. It is intended that subsequent editions will be more accurate than the current edition. Because mental health diagnoses are constructs, rather than absolutes, there will always be disagreements and inaccuracy. If a specific diagnosis was given for every possible mental health problem, there would be thousands, if not more, of diagnoses, because each would be somewhat different. Even in the most recent *DSM,* the *DSM-IV-TR,* several of the diagnoses are similar and often confused between professionals (e.g., Dysthymia vs. Chronic Adjustment Disorder, with Depression, or Major Depressive Disorder, with Psychotic Features vs. Schizoaffective Disorder).

It would be unwise and confusing to define a new diagnosis each and every time someone's symptoms vary from someone else's. Thus, when making a diagnosis, the clinician selects a diagnosis that is the best fit to the client. The closer the fit, the more valid the diagnosis. Many diagnoses are symptomatically composed of endorsing at least the minimal number of symptoms out of a select list. Thus, clients with the same diagnoses may have a number of symptoms in common and some not in common. Without this system there would have to be a separate diagnosis for every combination of symptoms.

Just as the color designated as *blue* is a description of a wide array of hues and not a specific wavelength of light, a *DSM-IV-TR* diagnosis suggests a general category that aids in communication between professionals, rather than an exact description. The *DSM-IV-TR* allows for clinical judgment in making a diagnosis when the individual does not clearly meet the diagnostic criteria, but the clinician believes that the diagnosis is warranted.

The *DSM-IV-TR* follows a common format for classifying disorders. Although some *DSM-IV-TR* disorders contain additional headings, the following is the basic outline for each:

Common DSM-IV-TR *Disorder Classification Headings*

> Code number
>
> Name of diagnosis
>
> Diagnostic features
>
> Associated features and disorders
>
>> Associated descriptive features and mental disorders
>>
>> Associated laboratory findings
>
> Specific age and gender features
>
> Prevalence
>
> Course
>
> Familial pattern
>
> Differential diagnosis
>
> Diagnostic criteria

ESSENTIAL SYMPTOMS

Essential symptoms of a diagnosis are symptoms that must be present to make a diagnosis. These symptoms are listed in the Diagnostic Features section for each *DSM-IV-TR* diagnosis. For example, the *DSM-IV-TR* (APA, 2000) lists the essential features of Dysthymic Disorder as, "a chronically depressed mood that occurs for most of the day more days than not for at least 2 years (children, 1 year), (Criterion A)" (p. 376). If an adult has felt depressed most of the time for only 1 year, the diagnosis is not Dysthymic Disorder. Also, the diagnosis cannot be made if the adult has been depressed 2 or more years, but only sporadically. Other essential symptoms are listed, but not all are required to be present to validate the diagnosis.

Primary and Secondary Essential Symptoms

The terms *primary essential symptoms* and *secondary essential symptoms* are not found in the literature but are used in this text to more clearly differentiate between two discrete types of essential symptoms. Some *DSM-IV-TR* classifications break down essential symptoms into two types but do not define them. The first includes symptoms (hereby referred to as *primary essential symptoms*) that must be present to validate a diagnosis. The *DSM-IV-TR* lists these symptoms first under the heading "Diagnostic Features." The second type includes symptoms (hereby referred to as *secondary essential symptoms*) of which only a certain number must be present to validate the diagnosis. The *DSM-IV-TR* combines both types, referring to them interchangeably as *essential symptoms*. Every *DSM-IV-TR* diagnosis features primary essential symptoms, but not all list secondary essential symptoms.

For example, to diagnose a client with Conduct Disorder, the client must exhibit the essential symptom of "a repetitive and persistent pattern of behavior in which the basic rights of others or major age-appropriate societal norms or rules are violated" (*DSM-IV-TR*, APA, 2000, p. 93). Other *DSM-IV-TR* disorders include both primary and secondary essential symptoms. In this case, the client must exhibit the primary symptom(s) but only exhibit a certain number (dictated by the *DSM-IV-TR*) of the other essential symptoms listed (secondary essential symptoms). For example, the *DSM-IV-TR* criteria for Oppositional Defiant Disorder (313.81) include primary essential symptoms of a recurrent pattern of negativistic, defiant, disobedient, and hostile behavior toward authority figures that persists for at least 6 months. In addition, during this period, four or more of the following secondary essential symptoms must be validated: "(1) often loses temper, (2) often argues with adults, (3) often actively defies or refuses to comply with adults' requests or rules, (4) often deliberately annoys people, (5) often blames others for his or her mistakes or misbehavior, (6) is often touchy or easily annoyed by others, (7) is often angry or resentful, (8) is often spiteful or vindictive" (pp. 102). Each of the validated symptoms must result in disturbance in behavior that causes clinically significant impairment in social, academic, or occupational functioning.

In the previous example, eight secondary essential symptoms of Oppositional Defiant Disorder are listed, but only four or more must be present, along with the primary essential symptom, to validate the symptoms of a diagnosis. It is, therefore, possible that two people with the same diagnosis could have no overlap in secondary essential symptoms. Even people with the same symptoms could experience different functional impairment. Thus, it is important to ensure that a diagnosis is documented carefully so that the treatment plan can be tailored to the individual client. A treatment plan that addresses a generic Oppositional Defiant Disorder diagnosis is not individually targeted and may not successfully return the client to normal functioning.

ASSOCIATED SYMPTOMS

Associated symptoms are symptoms present in or attributable to a diagnosis but not essential to formulating the diagnosis. They are often vegetative symptoms (e.g., weight loss, insomnia, and diminished libido [Maxmen & Ward, 1995]). The *DSM-IV-TR* lists various associated symptoms for most diagnoses. These symptoms are not used to validate a diagnosis but provide useful information for planning treatment and understanding the nature of the client's issues. Associated symptoms within a given diagnosis can vary among individuals. Symptoms not specifically listed in the *DSM-IV-TR* but that contribute to the client's functional impairments of a valid diagnosis may be added to the treatment plan.

Figure 5.1 describes the various symptoms associated with Dysthymic Disorder. According to the *DSM-IV-TR* (APA, 2000), the first essential symptom (primary essential symptom #1) must be present, along with two or more other essential symptoms (secondary essential symptoms #2–#7) to validate a diagnosis. Several associated symptoms (#1–#6) may also be present but are not necessary to justify the diagnosis.

Associated symptoms provide more information specifically about the client's situation. In this case, if the symptom in criterion A were present along with all of the symptoms in criteria C, yet no symptoms from criteria B were evident, *DSM-IV-TR* does not allow the diagnosis. (However, the *DSM-IV-TR* does allow for clinical judgment in making a diagnosis when an insufficient number of symptoms are endorsed.)

To validate the diagnosis in Figure 5.1, the clinician should first document criteria A and then document at least two of the symptoms listed in criteria B. The clinician may also document any symptoms from criteria C, although these do not need to be present to diagnose the disorder. In addition to documenting these symptoms, the clinician must elicit information regarding how these effects of Dysthymic Disorder are impairing either socially, occupationally, or in other areas of the client's life causing distress.

This book follows the *DSM-IV-TR*'s definition of essential and associated symptoms; however, this book differentiates between the two types of essential symptoms listed in the *DSM-IV-TR* by

FIGURE 5.1
DSM-IV-TR Symptoms of Dysthymic Disorder

A. *Primary Essential Symptoms*
(Necessary to validate a diagnosis)

1. Depressed most of day, for more days than not, as indicated either by subjective account or observation by others, for at least 2 years; and

B. *Secondary Essential Symptoms*
Presence, while depressed, of two or more of the following in order to validate a diagnosis

2. Poor appetite or overeating

3. Insomnia or hypersomnia

4. Low energy or fatigue

5. Low self-esteem

6. Poor concentration or difficulty making decisions

7. Feelings of hopelessness

C. *Associated Symptoms*
(Not sufficient to validate a diagnosis, but typically associated with the diagnosis)

1. Feelings of inadequacy

2. Generalized loss of interest or pleasure

3. Social withdrawal

4. Feelings of guilt or brooding about the past

5. Subjective feelings of irritability or excessive anger

6. Decreased activity, effectiveness, or productivity

Source: DSM-IV-TR (2000, pp. 376–378).

calling them *primary essential symptoms* and *secondary essential symptoms.* In the example of Dysthymic Disorder symptoms (Figure 5.1), the *DSM-IV-TR* combines the primary and secondary essential symptoms, referring to them as essential symptoms. The diagnostic portion of the initial interview is designed to rule in and rule out clinical syndromes. Crucial information is provided for clinical dialogue, treatment planning, and third-party review. The information gathered in the initial interview drives the treatment plan; therefore, it must be clinically specific.

During the diagnostic interview, the clinician should ask specific questions to validate the symptoms and criteria of a diagnosis. This process of ruling in and ruling out often accounts for as much as 30% to 40% of the interview time. As noted previously, it is crucial to ask questions regarding the onset, frequency, antecedents, intensity, and duration (OFAID procedure) of each symptom.

IMPAIRMENTS

Typically, when clients request mental health services, they suffer from dysfunction or impairments in their lives. They may have been exhibiting symptoms for a significant period of time without seeking services; however, when clients experience increasing dysfunction or impairments in their lives, the need for services becomes more pressing. That is, it is more common to hear a client in the initial interview make the statement, "My life is falling apart ... I might lose my job and family" (*impairments*), than to hear, "I am losing weight, not sleeping well, and I have low self-esteem" (*symptoms*). As symptoms increase in intensity, impairments become more apparent. One major difference between symptoms and impairments is that symptoms tend to be at a microlevel, affecting specific client behaviors, while impairments are more global, affecting major areas of the client's life. Endorsement of symptoms, without resulting impairments typically suggests that the level of symptoms is not at a level of severity in which services are medically necessary.

The *DSM-IV-TR* requires that clinically significant distress or impairment resulting in social, occupational, or other important areas of functioning exist before a diagnosis may be made. Examples of these impairments should be documented to validate the medical necessity for treatment. The level of impairment or dysfunction is a good indicator of the severity of symptoms.

EXAMPLES OF INTEGRATING DIAGNOSIS, SYMPTOMS, AND IMPAIRMENTS

Example 1

Cindy, age 24, has been diagnosed with Dysthymic Disorder (300.4; *diagnosis*). She describes the onset of her depression as 3 years ago when she moved out on her own. She feels depressed at least 75% of the time. There has never been more than a 2- to 3-week period in this time frame in which she has not felt depressed (*primary essen-*

tial symptoms). Ongoing symptoms include poor appetite, fatigue, and feelings of hopelessness (*secondary essential symptoms*). She further adds that she often isolates herself from others and doesn't want to do much but sit around the house (*associated symptoms*). She has never received another diagnosis of depression or mania, nor is her depression the result of a medical condition or substance abuse (*additional validation of diagnosis*). Prior to impairment she rarely missed work and surpassed her job quotas most of the time. Over the past 2 years, she has missed increasingly more work due to fatigue and low motivation. Last week she was given a warning at work due to absenteeism and significantly decreased productivity (*occupational impairment*). Prior to impairment, she was involved in sports teams and usually spent about 2 evenings per week with friends. Now she socializes about 1 evening per month, other than eating lunch daily with coworkers (*current functioning compared to previous functioning*). She describes herself as "lonely" and "not very interested in other people" (*social impairment*). She states that she "just feels numb" and doesn't care much about what happens in her future (*affective impairment*). Although she knows she must eat, she states that she is seldom hungry and has steadily lost about 5 to 10 pounds per year (*possible physical impairment*).

Example 2

Stephan C., age 7, is diagnosed with Attention-Deficit/Hyperactivity Disorder (ADHD), Predominantly Inattentive Type (314.00; *diagnosis*). He is described and observed by his parents, teacher, and school counselor as having persistent patterns of inattention significantly below what is expected for his level of development (*primary essential symptoms*). Observations by this examiner and review of records from his school and parents' collateral information indicate examples of symptoms of difficulties paying attention to details at home and school, poor attention span, lack of follow-through with homework or household chores, inability to keep track of possessions, and distractibility and forgetfulness during daily activities (*secondary essential symptoms*). He is reported to be prone to temper tantrums, stubbornness, and bossiness (*associated symptoms*). His parents first noticed most of these symptoms about the age of 4 or 5. Teachers began informing his parents of these issues in the first grade (*additional validation of diagnosis*). Although educational testing indicates a normal range of intellectual functioning, he is academically performing significantly below grade level. He is not learning age-appropriate material and has been referred to the Emotional/Behavioral Disorder (EBD) program at school (*educational impairment*). In school activities he is often ridiculed by his classmates for not paying attention. Subsequently, he has no friends and is often teased by his classmates, resulting in social withdrawal and low self-esteem (*social and affective impairment*).

THE RULE-IN/RULE-OUT PROCESS

The following illustration provides insight into the logic of the rule-in/rule-out process. If a man in Europe wanted directions to 5525 Main Street in North St. Paul, Minnesota in the United States, he would ask questions in a logical progression. That is, he should not ask, "Where is 5525, or where is 5525 Main Street?" because there are likely tens of thousands of 5525 Main Streets in the world. Instead, he should ask how to reach 5525 Main Street in North St. Paul, Minnesota in the United States. Thus, he is able to avoid going to several states or countries by asking where 5525 Main Street is located. A logical progression of questions avoids redundancy.

This illustration employs deductive rather than inductive methods of questioning, that is, moving from general to specific questioning to reach a conclusion. This principle holds true for the diagnostic interview as well. If a clinician asks information based on secondary essential and associated symptoms alone, it will be difficult to make a diagnosis because many *DSM-IV-TR* disorders have similar or related secondary and associated symptoms. For example, symptoms such as social withdrawal, low self-esteem, irritability, restlessness, fatigue, guilt, negativism, sleeping problems, weight changes, and poor concentration are clinically significant but are associated with several disorders including various types of depression, anxiety, Pain Disorders, and thought disorders. If the clinician only solicited information about these symptoms, it would be like asking how to find 5525 Main Street. The person may never get home or end up in the wrong place because the question wasn't specific. Diagnostically, misdirection may or may not become a litigious issue, but it certainly raises ethical and treatment issues.

A more efficient means of ruling in or ruling out a specific diagnosis is to first survey the primary essential symptoms of various *DSM-IV-TR* disorders. Interviewing clients concerning these symptoms differentiates the diagnostic categories, is time efficient, elim-

FIGURE 5.2
Poor Example of Rule-In/Rule-Out Process

T: Do you feel tired at times?

C: Yes.

T: Are there times when you just want to be left alone?

C: Yes.

T: Does your self-esteem seem to drop when you feel down?

C: You hit the nail on the head.

T: Do you feel uptight when you are under stress?

C: That's exactly it!

T: Is it harder to cope when you are under stress?

C: Yes. You seem to know exactly how I feel.

---

inates redundancy, and covers the spectrum of disorders. Figure 5.2 demonstrates a poor example of ruling in or ruling out specific disorders.

Although the dialogue in Figure 5.2 may suggest therapist empathy for the client's problem, it provides little diagnostic information. If the therapist assumes that the client's responses to the questions suggest Dysthymic Disorder, it may be accurate, but several other diagnoses have not been ruled out. For example, the symptoms endorsed in Figure 5.2 could suggest other *DSM-IV-TR* diagnoses as well, including any Depressive Disorder, an Adjustment Disorder, various Personality Disorders, or fatigue.

Even a person with no clear mental health diagnosis who is undergoing normal life stressors might complain of these symptoms. In this case, the Barnum Effect (Klopfer, 1960), in which overdiagnosis is possible due to vague specification of symptoms, is clearly evident. The therapist is asking questions that a majority of people, with or without psychopathology, would endorse. The client believes that the therapist is right on target. But diagnostically there is no clear target! That is because the therapist is using an inductive rather than a deductive model of questioning.

Figure 5.3 illustrates a better approach to diagnostic questioning but still does not produce a definitive diagnosis. The clinical questions in Figure 5.3 have more direction than Figure 5.2, but the questions are posed randomly. In this case, the client acknowledged feelings of depression and anxiety, but the clinician did not determine their effects, significance, or relationship with the presenting

FIGURE 5.3
Better, But Still Insufficient Example of Diagnosing a Disorder

---

T: Do you feel sad often?

C: Yes.

T: Are you often anxious?

C: Yes.

T: Do you ever have panic attacks?

C: No.

T: Have you been avoiding people lately?

C: I think so.

---

problem. Eventually these questions will have to be repeated and more specific information requested.

A better way to solicit client information and approach a diagnosis is to use the rule-in/rule-out process. The *DSM-IV-TR* is divided into 17 diagnostic categories (Figure 5.4). Each of the diag-

FIGURE 5.4
DSM-IV-TR Diagnostic Categories

---

1) Disorders Usually First Diagnosed in Infancy, Childhood, or Adolescence

2) Delirium, Dementia, and Amnestic and Other Cognitive Disorders

3) Mental Disorders Due to a General Medical Condition

4) Substance-Related Disorders

5) Schizophrenia and Other Psychotic Disorders

6) Mood Disorders

7) Anxiety Disorders

8) Somatoform Disorders

9) Factitious Disorders

10) Dissociative Disorders

11) Sexual and Gender Identity Disorders

12) Eating Disorders

13) Sleep Disorders

14) Impulse-Control Disorders Not Elsewhere Classified

15) Adjustment Disorders

16) Personality Disorders

17) Other Conditions That May Be a Focus of Clinical Attention

---

nostic categories contains diagnostic features unique from other categories. The rule-in/rule-out process allows the clinician to target information gathering and determine what information should be pursued and what is not as important, based on the client's reported symptoms and observable signs.

The clinician rarely needs to systematically go through all 17 (*DSM-IV-TR,* 2000, Table of Contents) diagnostic categories for each client. The nature of the client's presenting problem nearly always directs the focus of the interview. For example, a client who initially presents with complaints of depressed mood most likely is suffering from a Mood Disorder. As the interview progresses, it becomes clear if concerns in other areas not initially presented by the client also exist.

STEPS OF RULE-IN/RULE-OUT PROCESS

STEP ONE: Rule-In/Rule-Out Primary Essential Symptoms

Let's return to John Doe's intake session. The therapist asks a series of questions designed to rule in or rule out different categories of *DSM-IV-TR* disorders. Keep in mind that the therapist already ruled out a substance abuse problem earlier in the interview.

First, the therapist reviews the client's presenting problem.

T: You stated before that you are here because of depression.
JD: Yes, I've felt that way too many times in my life.
T: Have you ever been treated for any other mental health concerns?
JD: Just for the depression with Dr. Wilson five years ago that I told you about.
T: Are there any other concerns besides depression?
JD: I don't think so. The depression is bad enough.

The next questions rule out the possibility that the client is suffering from an Anxiety Disorder.

T: How about anxiety?
JD: What do you mean?
T: Do you often worry excessively or feel nervous, restless, or panicky?

JD: No, not often. Every once in a while I worry, but no more than anyone else with financial problems.

T: Do you have any history of panic attacks?

JD: What do you mean?

T: Do you ever experience symptoms such as dizziness, chest pain, difficulties breathing, or feeling out of control?

JD: Oh, maybe once or twice in my life, but not to that extent. I guess I'm not a worrier.

Next, the therapist rules out Cognitive Disorders such as Delirium, Dementia, Amnesia, and so on. (Information from the MSE is also used to rule out these disorders.)

T: Do you have problems with memory or concentration, or have people made comments about this to you?

JD: No, not really. Actually, my memory and concentration are pretty good.

The therapist also wants to rule out physical conditions that might produce a mental disorder.

T: You stated before that you are in pretty good health. Have you noticed any changes in your health or physical condition lately?

JD: I get tired or fatigued more easily, but it's not that bad.

T: How long have you felt more fatigued?

JD: Probably since I realized how depressing things are for me. I think it's because I used to be so active, and now I just don't feel like it. I'll get over it.

Next, the therapist rules out Somatoform Disorders.

T: For most of your teen or adult life, have you had a history of concerns such as frequent headaches, stomach aches, nausea, diarrhea, or memory lapses?

JD: No, not more than anyone else. I've always been healthy.

The therapist also rules out Schizophrenia and other Psychotic Disorders.

T: Have you ever or do you ever hear voices, and no one is there?

JD: Oh no!

T: Do you ever see things that no one else sees?

JD: What do you mean?

T: Like shadows walking on the wall or images that no one else sees but you.

JD: No, nothing at all like that.

T: Do you ever experience any unusual body sensations, smells, tastes, or feelings?

JD: Not at all.

Now, the therapist rules out mania.

T: Are there times in which you feel full of energy, maybe have little or no need for sleep, and feel like you are on top of the world?

JD: I wish I felt that way . . . no, not at all.

The therapist then rules out dissociation.

T: Do you ever feel like you have left your body, or do you feel like you are someone else?

JD: Not at all. What you see is what you get!

T: Have you ever had times when it felt like you just were not there, but your body was going through the motions?

JD: No, never.

Next, the therapist rules out Eating Disorders.

T: Do you have any concerns in any of the following areas? Eating, such as throwing up, or eating too much or too little?

JD: My appetite is high, and I've gained weight, but I'm not throwing up or binge eating.

T: Have you had any eating problems in the past?

JD: When I get depressed I gain weight.

And the therapist rules out a sleeping disorder.

T: Do you have problems falling asleep, sleeping too much, or sleeping too little?

JD: Well, since my wife died I've been waking up about an hour earlier than I'd like, but I'm getting used to it.

T: Once you fall asleep do you have any problems with terrors, nightmares, or sleepwalking?

JD: No, I don't.

Next, the therapist rules out Sexual or Gender Identity Disorders.

T: Do you have any sexual concerns or problems with sexual behavior?
JD: I've had no sex life since my wife died, but there are no sexual
    problems.

The therapist also rules out Impulse-Control Disorders.

T: Are any of your behaviors difficult to control, or do they get out of
    hand?
JD: No, this is not a problem.
T: Are there any areas of your life in which others have told you that
    you spend too much time or effort?
JD: What do you mean?
T: Like gambling, drugs, alcohol, sexual behaviors, or even time on
    the computer . . . anything like that?
JD: No, not at all.

Finally, the therapist rules out Adjustment Disorders.

T: Have there been any other major stressors or changes in your life
    in the past six months that are difficult to cope with now?
JD: None that I can think of.

These diagnostic questions were designed to rule in or rule out
primary essential symptoms of most *DSM-IV-TR* disorders. Before
making a diagnosis, the therapist wanted to rule out other *DSM-IV-TR* disorders such as anxiety, panic attacks, cognitive issues, physical concerns, somatization, thought disorders, mania, dissociation,
Eating Disorders, sleeping problems, sexual issues, and adjustment problems.

Notice that the clinician did not ask detailed questions about
John Doe's depression, other than requesting a history of the problem and eliciting John Doe's concerns about it. At this point, the clinician strongly suspects a mood disorder and has ruled out most
other categories of *DSM-IV-TR* disorders.

STEP TWO: Rule-In/Rule-Out Secondary Essential Symptoms

The clinician believes that John Doe is suffering from a mood disorder and has ruled out nonmood disorders. But more specific in-

formation is needed to make a differential diagnosis. The next step is to rule in or rule out specific mood disorders, specifically a depressive disorder. The clinician ruled out a bipolar disorder during step one. The information collected earlier in the interview, as well as knowledge of specific *DSM-IV-TR* criteria of the various mood disorders, also will be helpful in making a diagnosis. Questions in step two focus on symptomology, onset, frequency, duration, and severity of John Doe's impairments. Next, the therapist incorporates the appropriate aspects of the OFAID technique to provide much more specific diagnostic information.

T: I would like to ask you some more questions about your sadness or depression.
JD: Go ahead.

First, the therapist questions how long John Doe has felt depressed (*onset*).

T: How long have you felt this way?
JD: All of my life. I've never really been happy. I've never really felt good about myself. I'm a failure . . . but I function . . . That's all I do. It's just that now things are building up, and I need help. My rut is deeper than usual.

The next questions seek to verify the diagnosis of a specific disorder (*differential diagnosis*).

T: Have there ever been any extended periods of time when you were not depressed, say for more than two months?
JD: No, none that I can remember. Sometimes when major life events are taking place, like my graduation or getting married, I've felt better for a few weeks or so, but this is unusual.
T: Tell me more about how the depression now is different than your usual mood.
JD: Like I said before, I'm usually able to function, but now I don't want to. I'm down and don't feel like getting up. There's too much pressure. I'm alone. No one cares. I feel like I'm bottoming out. It's like . . . what's the use?
T: It sounds like you are usually down on yourself and look at life as hopeless, but now things are much worse than usual.
JD: That's exactly what I'm saying.

Next, the therapist determines how often John Doe feels depressed (*frequency*).

T: How often do you feel down or depressed?
JD: I feel down about every day.
T: How often do you not feel depressed?
JD: Maybe once a week.
T: What is it like then?
JD: I feel almost normal . . . like I might get ahead someday. I go shopping and take care of the things I should have done the rest of the week.

Now the therapist needs to determine how long this most recent bout of severe depression has lasted (*most recent onset or cycling of symptoms*).

T: Since you have felt depressed, has there been a time in which symptoms became noticeably worse?
JD: Yes, at first after her death I was handling it, but it has been getting much worse lately.
T: How long has it been worse like this?
JD: Probably about two months.
T: And nothing happened out of the ordinary two months ago?
JD: No, things just kept building up, and I began giving up.
T: Is the feeling similar to when you received counseling from Dr. Anderson five years ago?
JD: Yes, but even worse . . . at least I was married then.

Next, the therapist clarifies John Doe's specific symptoms (*clarification of symptoms*).

T: Do you ever have thoughts of suicide or dying?
JD: Sometimes I think it would be better for everyone if I wasn't around. I've even thought of ways to die.
T: Do you have a plan for suicide?
JD: Oh no. I would never commit suicide . . . I believe in God . . . I couldn't . . . wouldn't . . . do it.
T: Are you sure?
JD: Yes, for certain, but thanks for asking.
T: How is your appetite?
JD: I eat and eat and eat. It's never been so bad. Just six months ago I weighed 160 pounds. Now I weigh almost 190.

T: Is there anything enjoyable in your life at this time?

JD: Yes, I do enjoy reading and watching movies. They seem to be an escape.

Now the therapist clarifies how depression is affecting John Doe (*clarification of impairments*).

T: Has your depression affected any other areas of your life?

JD: What do you mean?

T: For example, you mentioned that you are on probation at work due to excessive absences. When I ask, "Are there any other areas in your life that have been affected by your depression?" I mean areas such as your social life, your physical health, or your thinking.

JD: I sometimes don't pay attention to things, and people think I'm forgetful. It's probably because I just don't care.

T: Do you have these times of confusion or poor concentration only when you are depressed or at other times also?

JD: It's only when I'm the most depressed . . . maybe once or twice a month since I've been down. It's part of the reason I'm missing so much work. I'm afraid.

T: For most of your life have you done well or have you had difficulty making decisions?

JD: It's always been a real chore. I change my mind because I believe my decisions are wrong. I never really make up my mind.

T: Tell me more about your social life.

JD: What social life? In the past few months I haven't returned any phone calls. Like I said before, I don't even spend time with my best friend. I've become a recluse. I haven't felt like getting out. I wouldn't even know what to say to someone if I were introduced to someone new. What would I talk about . . . my life is about as boring as it gets.

With these questions, the therapist has successfully ruled in both Major Depressive Disorder and Dysthymic Disorder. Some of the symptoms and impairments were validated in the initial screening, whereas others were validated when the therapist explored symptoms of specific Mood Disorders. As you can see from the *DSM-IV-TR* description of essential symptoms (Figure 5.5), the diagnosis is valid for both disorders.

FIGURE 5.5
Diagnosing John Doe with Major Depressive Disorder and Dysthymic Disorder

Diagnosis #1   Major Depressive Disorder

Must exhibit symptom in Criteria #1 and at least four symptoms from Criteria #2.

Criteria Met (X)	*DSM-IV-TR Essential Symptoms Criteria*
	Criteria #1 (Primary Essential Symptom)
X	Usual depressed mood or lack of pleasure, continuously for two or more weeks, resulting in social, occupational, and affective impairment or distress.
	Criteria #2 (Secondary Essential Symptoms)
X	Weight gain of over 5% per month
X	Increased appetite
	Insomnia or hypersomnia
	Psychomotor agitation or retardation
X	Fatigue
X	Worthlessness or guilt
X	Poor concentration
X	Thoughts of death/suicide

Diagnosis #2   Dysthymic Disorder

Must exhibit symptom in Criteria #1 and at least two symptoms from Criteria #2.

Criteria Met (X)	*DSM-IV-TR Essential Symptoms Criteria*
	Criteria #1 (Primary Essential Symptom)
X	Depressed more days than not for at least two years
	Criteria #2 (Secondary Essential Symptoms)
X	Poor appetite or overeating
	Insomnia or hypersomnia
X	Low energy or fatigue
X	Low self-esteem
	Poor concentration or difficulty making decisions
X	Feelings of hopelessness
	Other *DSM-IV-TR* Criteria
X	Not symptom-free for more than two months in past two years
X	Disorder not better accounted for by other *DSM-IV-TR* conditions

STEP THREE: Determine Associated Symptoms

The previous two diagnoses of Dysthymic Disorder and Major Depression were ruled in during the interview via steps one and two. Now sufficient information is available for the treatment plan. Additional questions posed in the interview could include eliciting additional associated symptoms to aid in providing a more clear understanding of the client's issues. Clinicians may also focus on items of interest helpful within their school of thought. For example, those from a systems approach will focus on the role of the family and significant others, whereas those from a dynamic approach will show more interest in how the client's early environment has impacted the client's current state.

LIMITATIONS OF THE DIAGNOSTIC INTERVIEW

The diagnostic interview is subject to limitations of validity and reliability. It is as valid as the *DSM-IV-TR* is valid in its diagnostic categories; however, some *DSM-IV-TR* diagnoses are more valid than others. For example, some disorders, such as Major Depressive Disorder, list clear symptoms that must be evident to make a valid diagnosis. To justify the diagnosis, the clinician compares the client's symptoms to the symptoms listed under the specific disorder in the *DSM-IV-TR*. Thus, this diagnosis is not likely to arouse much disagreement among professionals because its symptoms are clear cut.

Other *DSM-IV-TR* disorders do not have such straightforward or discrete symptoms, and many disorders have overlapping symptoms with other disorders. In these cases, clinicians may disagree on a diagnosis based on seemingly minor points. Some examples of disorders that have overlapping symptoms, thereby limiting the validity of their diagnosis, include (a) Bipolar Disorder and Borderline Personality Disorder, (b) Schizoaffective Disorder and Major Depression with Psychotic Features, and (c) Major Depression; Mild, Recurrent Type, and Dysthymic Disorder, among others.

The reliability of a diagnostic interview depends on the clinician's knowledge of psychopathology and the consistency of the examination. The clinician should always ask clients the same general set of questions when ruling in or ruling out various disorders. When different sets of questions are posed to different clients, important diagnostic questions may be forgotten to be asked; thus, misdiagnosis could occur. Thorough knowledge of psychopathology and the *DSM-IV-TR* enables the clinician to stay on target. Memorizing specific symptoms of the major mental disorders is a crucial time-saving skill that enables the experienced clinician to quickly perform the rule-in/rule-out process.

This chapter has provided information to help formulate an accurate diagnosis. The next step to helping the client return to normal functioning is to formulate an individualized and detailed treatment plan.

HIGHLIGHTS
of Chapter 5

★ In order for a diagnosis to be validated, there must be a sufficient number of symptoms and resulting impairment to meet diagnostic criteria in the *DSM-IV-TR*. Both symptoms and impairments should be clearly documented throughout the course of therapy until the diagnosis is no longer prevalent.

★ The *DSM-IV-TR* diagnoses are broken down into essential and associated symptoms.

★ Essential symptoms are those which must be prevalent in order to give a diagnosis.

★ Associated symptoms do not validate a diagnosis but are often present when a diagnosis occurs.

★ Interviewing time can be more efficient when essential symptoms are determined before associated symptoms because most associated symptoms are common to several diagnoses.

★ The rule-in/rule-out process in diagnostic interviewing saves much time in the interview process by systematically validating the existence (or lack of) of *DSM-IV-TR* essential and associated symptoms and the subsequent diagnosis.

★ The mere existence of symptoms does not validate mental health problems unless they are significantly impairing to the individual.

★ The diagnostic interview is limited by both its validity and reliability.

QUESTIONS

1. Which of the following interview questions best represents potential problems due to the Barnum Effect?

    (a) "Do you experience auditory hallucinations when you are severely depressed?"

    (b) "Does your level of depression cause you to miss a significant amount of work?"

    (c) "How long do your panic attacks generally last?"

    (d) "Do you get upset when you don't get your way?"

2. The diagnostic interview incorporates a procedure in which the client is asked whether he or she is experiencing various symptoms. Deciding on the subsequent questions is determined by the answers to the earlier questions. This process is called

    (a) rule-in/rule-out.

    (b) symptoms evaluations.

    (c) backtracking.

    (d) goal development.

3. Which of the following descriptors of behaviors are suggested in the text as helpful in determining both a specific diagnosis and level of functional impairments?

    (a) essential and associated symptoms

    (b) diagnosis and treatment

    (c) treatment plan, progress notes, discharge summary

    (d) onset, frequency, antecedents, intensity, and duration

4. What is clearly wrong with the following statement? "Pat endorses symptoms of social withdrawal, low motivation, low self-esteem, sleeping problems, and irritability; therefore, she meets criteria for Dysthymic Disorder."

    (a) The symptoms do not match that of a person with the diagnosis.

    (b) The essential symptoms criteria is not met.

    (c) No associated symptoms are mentioned.

    (d) All of the above.

Answers: 1. d; 2. a; 3. d; 4. b

6

Treatment Planning

Why treatment planning? It is accountability, clarity, communication, compensation, competency, compliance, consistency, dialogue, direction, documentation, ethics, evaluation, focus, goals, integration, justification, measurement, monitoring, needs, objectives, planning, preferences, record keeping, standardization, strategies, strengths, symptoms, and validation.

Treatment plan writing in the mental health field is a relatively recent development. Prior to the 1970s, formalized treatment plans were not part of the mental health delivery system. Early treatment plans provided little information other than vague acknowledgments that psychotherapy would occur. As managed care and accrediting agencies have increased the requirements for clinical efficacy, the quality of treatment plans has improved. The advent of managed care and regulatory agencies such as CARF, JCAHO, Champus, and Medicare have led to increasingly stringent accountability procedures; therefore, detailed treatment planning is now an important part of the therapeutic process. Currently, regulatory agencies and third-party payers have similar requirements in treatment plan writing.

A survey conducted by this author of more than 2,000 mental health professionals revealed that less than 3% of currently practicing mental health professionals (e.g., psychologists, social workers, Licensed Marriage and Family Therapists (LMFTs), and counselors) were formally trained or supervised in accountability procedures, such as treatment plan and progress note writing. A myriad of texts have been written about mental health treatment and how to conduct therapy, but few teach how to write and follow treatment plans or document the course of therapy.

COMPUTERIZED TREATMENT PLANNING

Siegel and Fischer (1981) noted that the treatment plan is the most frequently consulted portion of a client's chart. One of the biggest complaints about writing detailed treatment plans is the time it takes to develop them (Galasso, 1987; Ormiston, Barrett, Binder, & Molyneux, 1989; Walters, 1987). Luckily, research in computerized treatment planning has flourished, and computer-generated treatment plans have become an effective and time-saving resource to clinicians.

Some early computer programs developed "canned" treatment plans that were designed to fit *DSM* criteria for various diagnoses; however, they did not provide for the client's individual needs or the alleviation of functional impairments. Some facilities use these treatment plans with potentially disastrous results. For example, a therapist might diagnose a client with Dysthymic Disorder and then pull out a "Dysthymia Treatment Plan" from a packet of several diagnostic choices. To begin treatment, the therapist fills in the client's name and signs the prewritten plan. Although treatment plans of this variety are better than no treatment plan, they are designed to address global symptoms of a diagnosis and ignore the client's special needs and desires. These types of plans do not allow the therapist to develop a collaborative and individualized plan for treating specific clients who may have unique symptoms and impairments.

Widespread accepted standards and language in treatment plan writing is developing, however, and computer software development over the past 10 to 15 years has provided some promising solutions. Today's computerized treatment plans have added increasingly more options for the therapist to individualize treatment. The Thera*Scribe*® 4.0 treatment planning software (Wiley, 2004) has received positive reviews because it allows the clinician to customize the course of treatment based on the client's needs, and it follows current guidelines. It is user-friendly and saves considerable time in the writing process.

Little has been published that demonstrates *how* to write treatment plans with measurable and observable objectives that meet current managed care criteria other than the guidelines for each agency. This chapter shows how to integrate current agency and managed care requirements into properly documented, individualized treatment plans.

GETTING STARTED

Treatment plan objectives should be formulated to alleviate a client's functional impairments resulting from symptoms of a *DSM-IV-TR* disorder. It is important that treatment plans be designed to address the client's needs, rather than simply the diagnosis.

Writing treatment plans is easiest for clinicians who are thoroughly knowledgeable with the *DSM-IV-TR* and competent in diagnostic interviewing techniques. Excellent texts that integrate both areas include Othmer and Othmer's *The Clinical Interview Using DSM-IV-TR* (2002), Groth-Marnat's *Handbook of Psychological Assessment* (2003), and Morrison's DSM-IV *Made Easy* (1995).

TREATMENT PLAN DEVELOPMENT

Both a poor and an excellent treatment plan take relatively the same amount of time to write. Actually, a writer with little or improper training in treatment plan writing may take significantly more time to write the plan than a trained writer. Sufficient training and understanding of treatment plan writing enables one to write an effective treatment plan in a brief time period, in the session with the client, and with results that are therapeutic to the client and in compliance with third-party requirements.

Typically, the treatment plan is written in the second session with the client. The therapist goes over the diagnostic information collected in the initial session and collaborates with the client as to what impairments will be addressed in treatment.

An individualized treatment plan is based on detailed and accurate clinical information that corresponds with the client's strengths, weaknesses, abilities, and preferences (SNAPs) plus symptoms and respective functional impairments. Treatment plans formulate strategies to alleviate these impairments by incorporating client variables that would result in the most effective treatment. The chance of misdiagnosis and unresponsive treatment increases if essential symptoms, resulting impairments, and other client variables are not validated or incorporated into the treatment plan.

Historically, third-party payers have focused on the Axis I diagnoses as the primary determinant for reimbursement and the number of authorized sessions. Today, nearly all third-party payers still require an Axis I mental health diagnosis before authorizing for mental health services; moreover, there is a trend to exclude reimbursement for a growing number of specific Axis I diagnoses (e.g., Conduct Disorder, NOS diagnoses, and Adjustment Disorders). It is important for therapists to familiarize themselves with the specific authorization procedures and any exceptions for receiving services of each third-party payer. There are times in which it is possible to receive authorization for services when a diagnosis is not covered, but the documentation demonstrates medical necessity of services.

Reimbursement for services is most affected by the degree of functional impairment resulting from the mental disorder. Treatment handbooks, such as Roth and Fonagy's *What Works for Whom?* (2004) and Barlow's *Clinical Handbook of Psychological Disorders* (2001), provide information regarding the average number of visits and types of therapy indicated for various disorders; however, the diagnosis itself does not determine the level of mental health services needed. For example, it is possible for two people to be diagnosed with the same disorder but exhibit different levels of impairment. Other factors could impact these individuals' functioning, including history, personality, social supports, genes, and life stressors, among others. For two people with the same diagnosis, one might receive therapy to return to normal functioning, whereas the other could decompensate. One of the several purposes of the diagnostic interview is to document this information and provide appropriate treatment recommendations.

A well-thought-out treatment plan addresses the individual's strengths and limitations. It goes beyond diagnosis, symptoms, and impairments. Responding only to *DSM-IV-TR* symptoms may be technically correct but may not meet a client's therapeutic needs. This book described earlier how to solicit and clearly document detailed examples of a client's level of functioning and contributing factors to mental health concerns in the initial interview. Although symptoms and functional impairments are similar concepts, fundamental differences exist. Symptoms are distinct terms by which a mental or physical disorder is defined, whereas impairments are problem areas or functional limitations in the client's life that are adversely affected by the symptoms.

The client's strengths, needs, abilities, and preferences (SNAPs) should be accounted for in the treatment plan. The Joint Commission of Accreditation of Healthcare Organizations requires that the client actively participate in designing the treatment plan. Similar to building a house from a blueprint, both the buyer (client) and architect (therapist) work together to develop a mutually satisfying product. When people build a home, most have a fairly good idea of what they want it to look like. Likewise, many, but not all, people entering therapy have an idea of what they want to accomplish. Therefore, the architect (therapist) does not simply hand them a plan and say, "Here is your plan." Rather, they provide helpful guidance, based on their training and experience, in which they consider the strengths and limitations of the buyer's (client's) ideas. Together they will develop a realistic and workable plan within reach of the client and within the expertise of the therapist.

Third-party requirements can also affect treatment plan development. For example, third parties often limit the number of sessions per year they will reimburse. Thus, if the insurance company limits reimbursement to 12 sessions per year and the client is unable to pay for additional sessions, the treatment plan should be written to realistically utilize the 12 allotted sessions and provide for closure for the treatment at the end of session 12. If the client needs additional sessions, the therapist should help the client obtain them either through a request for additional services or by other means available.

Situational variables should also be considered when planning treatment. For example, if a client will only commit to 2 months of therapy because of an impending move, the treatment plan should be realistic, given this limitation. Lofty goals will lead to an unfulfilled course of therapy.

GOALS AND OBJECTIVES

Goals are the desired outcomes of therapy, and *objectives* are incremental steps used to accomplish treatment plan goals. Without specific goals and objectives to provide direction, treatment may be vague and lack direction. Measurable and observable objectives allow the therapist and client to evaluate the effectiveness of interventions, client progress, level of treatment, and the appropriate time of termination. In addition, regular evaluation of the client's progress toward goals can serve as a motivator for the client to stay on target with treatment issues. Effective treatment plans answer the questions, "Why am I in therapy?" "What will we talk about and do?" "How do I know how well therapy is working?" and "How will we know when therapy should terminate?" Progress notes, which will be discussed in Chapter 7, document that the treatment plan is being followed.

A number of publications and agencies recommend guidelines for developing treatment plans. For example, the *Standards for Behavioral Healthcare* (JCAHO, 2004) presents standards for mental

FIGURE 6.1
Overview of CARF (2004) Standards for Treatment Planning (Individual Plan)

1. The individual plan is developed with the active participation of the persons served, and:
   a. Is prepared using the information from the primary assessment and interpretive summary.
   b. Is based on the needs and desires of the persons served and focuses on his or her integration and inclusion into:
      (1) The local community.
      (2) The family, when appropriate.
      (3) Natural support systems.
      (4) Other services needed.
   c. Involves the family of the person served, when applicable or permitted.
   d. Identifies any needs beyond the scope of the program.
   e. Specifies the services to be provided by the program.
   f. Specifies referrals for additional services.
   g. Is communicated to the person served in a manner that is understandable.
   h. When possible, is provided to the person served.
   i. Is reviewed periodically with the person served for continuing relevance as is modified as needed.
2. The individual plan contains the following components:
   a. Goals that are:
      (1) Expressed in the words of the person served.
      (2) Reflective of the informed choice of the person served or parent/guardian.
      (3) Appropriate to the person's culture.
      (4) Appropriate to the person's age.
      (5) Based on the person's:
         (a) Strengths.
         (b) Needs.
         (c) Abilities.
         (d) Preferences.
   b. Specific service or treatment objectives that are:
      (1) Reflective of the expectations of:
         (a) The person served.
         (b) The treatment team.
      (2) Reflective of the client's expectations.
      (3) Reflective of the person's development.
      (4) Reflective of the person's culture and ethnicity.
      (5) Reflective of the person's disabilities/disorders or concerns.

FIGURE 6.1 (Continued)

(6) Understandable to the person served.

(7) Measurable.

(8) Achievable.

(9) Time specific.

(10) Appropriate to the treatment setting.

c. Frequency of specific treatment interventions.

d. Information on, or conditions for, transition to other services.

e. When applicable, identification of:

(1) Legal requirements.

(2) Legally imposed fees.

4. Signed and dated progress notes document:

a. Completion of the individual plan.

b. Significant events or changes in the life of the person served.

c. The delivery of services that support the individual plan.

5. A designated individual(s) in coordinating services for each person served by:

a. Assuming responsibility for ensuring the implementation of the individual plan.

b. Ensuring that the person served is oriented to his or her services.

c. Promoting the participation of the person served on an ongoing basis in discussions of his or her plans, goals, and status.

d. Identifying and addressing gaps in the service provision.

e. Sharing information on how to access community resources relevant to his or her needs.

f. Advocating for the person served, when applicable.

g. Communicating information regarding progress of the person served to the appropriate persons.

h. Facilitating the transition process, including arrangements for follow-up services.

i. Involving the family or legal guardian, when applicable or permitted.

j. Coordinating services provided outside of the organization.

k. Identifying the process for after-hours contact.

Source: Used by permission of the Behavioral Health Standards Manual. Commission on Accreditation of Rehabilitation Facilities. Copyright 2004.

health services, including assessment, treatment planning, time frames, and discharge status. The CARF treatment plan standards are listed in Figure 6.1. Medicare also has guidelines for clinicians to follow when preparing treatment plans and requires plans to include both long-range and short-range goals (Medicare, 1984).

The therapist and client work together to establish treatment goals. Therapeutic interventions, treatments, or strategies are not goals; rather, they are the therapeutic means by which the goals and objectives will be achieved. Part of the intake process should include discussing what changes the client would like to make and how they might be accomplished. Some treatment strategies designed to accomplish the client's goals are implemented in the session and others are implemented outside the session (e.g., homework or referrals).

In most cases, goals should reflect the alleviation of unwanted symptoms by attaining positive functional behaviors. The Joint Commission of Accreditation of Healthcare Organizations requires that treatment plan goals be linked to living, learning, and work activities. In addition, objectives should be written in observable, measurable terms so that outcomes can be evaluated impartially. For example, the goal "increase positive social interactions" might be achieved through specific objectives (attained by the client) such as "attend one social function per week" or "attend weekly social skills group meeting." Treatment strategies might include therapist interventions such as "positive reinforcement of target behaviors" or "role playing means of meeting new people."

Treatment plans are revised as the client progresses in meeting objectives. The JCAHO standards indicate that treatment goals should be periodically evaluated and revised. The Joint Commission of Accreditation of Healthcare Organizations does not impose a specific time frame for periodic evaluation; however, managed care companies often require treatment plan revisions after a set number of sessions or a given time period, such as every 3 months, every 6 to 10 sessions, or whenever best suits the client's needs.

A key factor to ensuring the client's successful accomplishment of objectives is how they are written. When objectives are either too simple or too difficult, clients will not be appropriately motivated to accomplish them. For example, extremely low expectations or easy objectives provide the client with little motivation to change behavior. Overly high expectations, on the other hand, can produce anxiety, resulting in the client's avoidance of the objective targets.

Likewise, vague and unclear objectives may lead to lengthy treatment but provide little or no direction regarding how they will help the client reach treatment goals, thereby reducing the probability of behavioral change. The obvious problem of establishing vague objectives such as "increase social interactions" is the difficulty in demonstrating significant change. For example, because the word *increase* is not quantified, even a change of .001% implies

FIGURE 6.2
Revising Objectives to Reach Targeted Goals: Increase Social Interactions

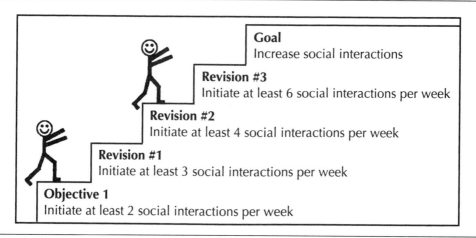

Goal
Increase social interactions

Revision #3
Initiate at least 6 social interactions per week

Revision #2
Initiate at least 4 social interactions per week

Revision #1
Initiate at least 3 social interactions per week

Objective 1
Initiate at least 2 social interactions per week

attainment of the objective. Change of this magnitude will most likely not significantly change the client's level of impairment. Specific objectives clarify progress in treatment. Thus, clearly written treatment plan objectives that require a moderate amount of effort to achieve provide the greatest probability of success.

As noted, treatment plans are not static. As objectives are accomplished, they are revised to more closely reach the stated goal. If each objective is a step toward the goal, then the last objective best reflects the goal (Goodman, Brown, & Dietz, 1996). This does not mean that every change in a treatment plan requires a new form to be filled out. Incremental revisions may be noted in progress notes, and the treatment plan only revised as necessary (e.g., as required by third parties or institutional policies or when writing a prior authorization request). Treatment plans extend for a specified period or number of sessions after which they are to be revised to reflect therapeutic progress.

The timing of treatment and the number of steps needed to accomplish treatment goals are highly related to the client's degree of impairment. Figure 6.2 depicts the relationship between goals and objectives by illustrating how incrementally more challenging objectives will help a client reach a target number of initiated social interactions. Figure 6.3 features objectives that demonstrate incremental steps toward a goal of systematic desensitization to airline travel. Although a treatment plan would not be rewritten every time an objective is reached, the progress notes could document revisions to it.

FIGURE 6.3
Revising Objectives to Reach Targeted Goal: Systematic Desensitization to Airplane Travel

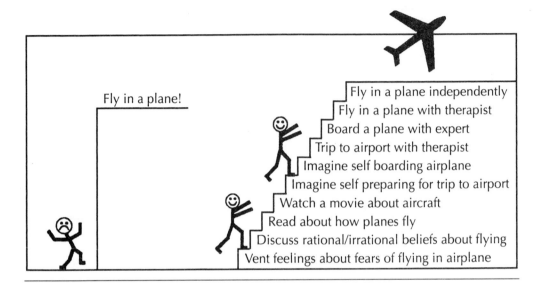

Figures 6.2 and 6.3 illustrate how incremental objectives are used to help clients reach a goal. If, for example, the client in Figure 6.2 was initially given the objective of flying in a plane, it might be overwhelming. Incremental objectives allow the client to gradually make therapeutic progress.

Other variables, such as the client's motivation, insight, and cooperation and rapport with the therapist, as well as the therapist's clinical skills, must be considered in the timing of treatment plan objectives. In many managed care settings in which the number of sessions is limited, time becomes a precious commodity.

Cognitive dissonance (tension caused by a conflict between one's established beliefs/attitudes/behaviors vs. opposing beliefs/attitudes/behaviors) often occurs when the therapist's training does not match current third-party documentation requirements. The dissonance often results in stress, discomfort, complaining, and worrying. It can be reduced when specific training and experience in current documentation and time-limited therapeutic procedures are provided. The dissonance often stems from the stress induced from lack of training; therefore, additional training will help change the therapist's attitude and behaviors.

TREATMENT PLAN REQUIREMENTS OF THIRD-PARTY PAYERS

Third-party payers, such as insurance companies and managed care providers, have their own rules and regulations regarding development and maintenance of treatment plans. Figure 6.4 depicts common requirements.

BEHAVIORAL OBJECTIVES: MEASURABLE AND OBSERVABLE

Terms such as *measurable* and *observable,* as required by managed care companies and regulatory agencies, follow the scientific-practitioner model, in which empirical or observable evidence is crucial to outcomes. Vague treatment plans, for example, might include an unclear objective such as, "increase communication skills." In this case the concept of communication skills is not clear. The term *communicate* might be interpreted as anything from a client's poor speech patterns to his or her ability to express emotions. Specificity is needed. In addition, because the objective is stated in relative terms, measurement is evasive. As noted earlier, objectives incorporating words such as *increase, decrease, add, change,* and so

FIGURE 6.4
Third-Party Payer Requirements for Treatment Plan Development and Maintenance

Competence: The service provider must have appropriate credentials to perform the indicated type of service and must be competent in the area of expertise for the particular mental disorder.

Medical Necessity: There must be documentation of dysfunction or functional impairment resulting from a mental disorder (defined in DSM or ICD) that significantly interferes with the client's activities of daily living.

Goals/Objectives: The treatment plan must include specific, attainable, observable, and measurable goals and objectives.

Treatment: Level and amount of treatment must be concordant with intensity of impairment. Type of treatment must be consistent with acceptable procedures that reliably predict outcomes. Treatment is directed toward the active signs of a disorder.

Ongoing Documentation: Progress notes must follow specific treatment plan objectives designed to alleviate functional impairments that have been clearly documented in the assessment and in the treatment plan.

on, with no further clarification, are vague because they do not quantify or give helpful direction to the degree of change.

It is suggested that the clinician first determine the symptoms of the disorder to formulate a *DSM-IV-TR* diagnosis and then question the client about functional impairments (e.g., social, occupational, physical) due to the effects of the mental health disorder. The clinician should then determine baseline measures for the functional impairments and set goals and incremental objectives for treatment.

It is difficult to measure and observe symptoms, but the resulting impairments are easily documented in a measurable manner. For example, documenting that a client is 75% depressed is a poor attempt to provide measurable evidence of impairment because the construct of depression is too vague to quantify. But the behavioral effects of depression can be quantified. For example, "The client misses school 75% of the time due to depression."

Subjective Units of Distress (SUDS)

The impact of symptoms can be estimated using Subjective Units of Distress (SUDs), which are measured on a scale of 1 to 100. Clients periodically are asked to rate their level of distress for variables such as anxiety, fear, depression, and so on. Clinicians who utilize this technique will ask clients to rate their SUD levels at the onset of therapy and then ask them to periodically reassess those levels as therapy progresses to evaluate the effects of treatment. The treatment plan can incorporate goals and objectives based on a client's SUD levels. For example, the treatment plan might state:

> Anxiety level when leaving the house. Current SUD: 90. Goal: 30. Four-week objective: 70.

Figure 6.5 illustrates a client's SUD using a graph.

VARYING BELIEFS AND PROCEDURES

Some therapeutic schools of thought claim that incorporating measurable outcomes contradicts their basic tenet of therapy. This statement might be true if measurable outcomes focused on symptoms rather than impairments. For example, many insight-oriented clinicians do not view therapeutic progress in terms of reducing symp-

FIGURE 6.5
Graphic Representation of Subjective Units of Distress (SUD)

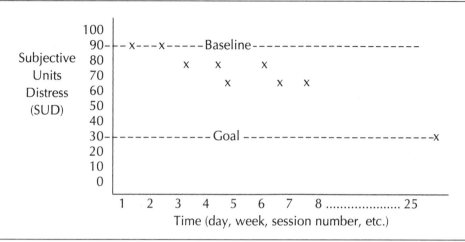

toms. They believe that "symptom substitution" will occur, that is, new symptoms emerge as others decline. They do not focus on symptoms because they believe that the underlying causes of the symptoms should be the focus of therapy. Therefore, a systematic measurement of symptoms becomes moot. Thus, advocates from a number of treatment modalities ask, "If we must validate a diagnosis with symptoms but do not believe that outcomes should be measured based on symptom changes, what else is there to measure?" To answer this question, it is necessary to point out that at least three processes take place in mental health treatment, regardless of the clinician's therapeutic orientation. These include (a) assessment, (b) treatment, and (c) discharge. Each part of treatment avails itself to different types of documentation.

Assessment

The assessment phase involves determining whether the client needs mental health services. That is, the clinician ascertains by various means the degree in which problem areas exist. A major point of the assessment is to validate the diagnosis of a disorder via symptoms and resulting impairments. No matter what theoretical orientation the therapist supports, certain criteria within the theoretical model are used to determine whether a client would benefit from mental health services. The same measures used to determine whether services are needed can also be used to determine when services are no longer necessary.

Treatment

The specific procedures in the treatment phase varies depending on which mode of therapy is used. The clinician documents changes in impairments throughout the course of therapy. Whether the clinician's type of treatment intends to modify behaviors, clarify cognitions, increase insight, or focus on the future is not important in documenting behavioral change. What matters is documenting that the treatment employed is alleviating the impairments that made treatment necessary.

Analogously, there are several means of traveling across the country, including, but not limited to, airplane, bus, automobile, motorcycle, bicycle, and walking. Although each mode of transportation is quite different, requiring different preparations, experiences, and time allotments, each will eventually get the person across the country. Nevertheless, the goal is to get across the country, which can be reached through a number of means. The various providers of transportation may disagree as to what mode is the best, but what matters is whether the person makes it across the country. Each transportation provider describes how the trip is made through their mode of transportation. Likewise, even though the mental health schools of thought might vary significantly in the preparations, experiences, and time allotments, they each intend to reach the client's original intention; reach the goal.

Discharge

If treatment goes a full course, it lasts until the client is able to adequately function in those areas that were previously impaired. Documentation is provided by regularly evaluating progress toward the goals of the treatment plan.

VALIDATING CHANGE

Validating changes in impairments is an easy documentation task compared to quantifying symptoms. The process of documenting a client's impairments is free from differences in therapeutic schools of thought because it is simply part of documenting a client's presenting problem and goals. During therapy, changes in these impairments can be achieved and measured by the objectives listed in the treatment plan. For example, the vague objective to "increase social interactions" could be revised to "initiate an average of two new social interactions per week by August 10th." When the client accomplishes this objective, it could be revised again to "initiate three social interactions per week by October 15th." Thus, the objective remains concrete and targeted, and the effectiveness of treatment is easily measured. How these objectives are achieved is not important from a documentation standpoint. For example, some therapists might use session time to teach the client to be more socially outgoing, whereas others might focus on the client's thought patterns. Still others may explore how the client's early life experiences influence his or her ability to interact with others. The treatment plan simply provides examples of behaviors for which changes will be documented to validate therapeutic progress.

A major point of documentation is to provide evidence of the effectiveness of treatment. Clinicians should be careful to select objectives that are consistent with their treatment methods. The probability of success is increased when the client is instrumental in formulating objectives.

Precautions must be taken against overmeasuring goals and objectives. Not all behaviors are measurable in clearly quantifiable terms; however, it is advisable to do so whenever possible. For example, it is difficult to quantify behaviors such as level of insight, respect for authority, level of self-esteem, mental confusion, and ability to concentrate.

INSIGHT-ORIENTED THERAPY AND TREATMENT PLANNING

Perhaps the most resistance to incorporating observable and measurable outcomes in treatment plans comes from therapists who conduct insight-oriented therapy, not due to problems with the treatment, but due to theoretical conflicts. Documenting level of insight is not clearly subject to quantification, plus the concept of symptoms reduction does not fit into the theoretical frame of reference. These clinicians find the medical model frame of reference incompatible with treating intrapsychic conflicts. Nevertheless,

FIGURE 6.6
Psychodynamic Target Areas in Treatment Plan Writing

Self-concept and identity

Low self-esteem/self confidence

Unclear/unstable identity/sense of self

Uncertain masculine/feminine identity

Self-concept and identity disrupted by dissociation

Interpersonal relationships

Excessive interpersonal isolation

Unstable relationships

Hypersensitivity to rejection and perceived abandonment

Inability to function autonomously

Excessive dependency

Continual perception of victimization/abuse/exploitation

Extreme distrust of others

Extreme hostility in interactions with others

Oppositionalism/indirect opposition to demands

Dishonest behavior

Extreme self-centeredness/arrogance

Hypersensitivity to criticism

Deficient social skills

Thinking and cognition

Impaired contact with reality

Disorganized thinking

Failure of accommodation to cognitive deficits

Flashbacks with confusion of past and present

Emotional functioning

Depressed mood

Suicidal intentions/preoccupation

Mood-related withdrawal from people/activities

Hyperactivity/euphoria

Tension/fearfulness/panic

Excessive and unrealistic guilt feelings

Mood swings

FIGURE 6.6 (Continued)

Impulse regulation/addiction

Impulsivity

Substance abuse (specify)

Self-injurious behavior

Violence

Flight/elopement

Inhibition/overcontrol

Adaptive skills

Impairment in activities of daily living

Impairment in academic/vocational skills

Poor medication compliance

Family

Lack of age-appropriate autonomy

Alienation from family

Marital difficulties

Parenting problems

Poor family alliance with treatment team

Other (including medical)

Source: J. G. Allen, J. R. Buskirk, and L. M. Sebastian (1992).

Gabbard (2000) notes that treatment plans are an integral part of the mental health service system just as psychodynamic theory is a major part of psychiatry; therefore, the two must be integrated.

Allen, Buskirk, and Sebastian (1992) discuss and provide examples of treatment plans developed at the Menninger Clinic in which therapists provide traditional psychodynamic treatment but document client progress in behavioral terms. Figure 6.6 represents typical psychodynamic target areas that can be documented in the listed behavioral terms. The authors provide eight problem domains of focus in Figure 6.7.

TYPES OF MEASUREMENT

There are four traditional types of data that can be measured: nominal, ordinal, interval, and ratio. In addition, a seldom-noted type of data, ordinal-metric (Wiger & Solberg, 2001) may be helpful in doc-

FIGURE 6.7
Example of Psychodynamic Treatment Plan

Example #1

Problem focus

Severe dissociation and discontinuity in identity associated with profoundly impaired interpersonal and vocational functioning. Manifested by amnesia, loss of job, propensity to be exploited by others, and inability to take care of basic needs.

Long-range goal

Patient will establish and maintain continuous self-awareness and develop a coherent sense of self.

Short-term goals (objectives)

1. Patient will report discontinuities in experience (amnesia) to self.
2. Patient will make a list of alter personalities and describe each.
3. Patient will initiate communication among alter selves.
4. Patient will identify alter personalities for staff.
5. Patient will keep a journal to record experience of alter personalities.
6. Patient will verbalize awareness of situations/feelings that trigger emergence of alter personalities.
7. Patient will take responsibility for actions.
8. Patient will verbalize understanding of the origins of his/her alter personalities/fugue states.

Example #2

Problem focus

Impaired contact with reality and extreme social isolation. Manifested by paranoid delusions, auditory hallucinations, inability to leave the house and to function at work, and deterioration of personal hygiene.

Long-range goal (a)

Patient's perception will be accurate.

Short-term goals (objectives)

1. Patient will take medication as prescribed and report effects.
2. Patient will plan and carry through a schedule of activities.
3. Patient will check out perceptions and assigned nursing/activity therapy staff.

Long-range goal (b)

Short-term goals (objectives)

1. Patient will compare beliefs with those of other patients.
2. Patient will discuss unrealistic beliefs and the psychological basis.

Source: J. G. Allen, J. R. Buskirk, and L. M. Sebastian (1992).

umentation. Behavioral objectives can incorporate nominal, ordinal, ordinal-metric, or interval data. There is no use for ratio data (requiring an absolute zero, which is not a behavioral concept); interval is the highest measure available in behavioral data. Nominal data in treatment objectives demonstrate whether a behavior takes place. Ordinal data suggest increases or decreases in behaviors but do not quantify the amount of behavioral change. Ordinal-metric data is a cross between ordinal and interval. Interval data allow the observer to determine the amount of behavioral change; thus, these data are more precise than ordinal data. Table 6.1 illustrates the various means by which objectives may be measured.

TREATMENT STRATEGIES

Treatment strategies incorporated in the treatment plan should reflect interventions that have been proven efficacious in the field. Clinicians should avoid including vague treatment strategies, such as individual therapy, because they do not adequately describe what interventions are taking place. Information in the treatment plan about specific interventions should include (a) type of therapy (e.g., individual, group, or family), (b) school of thought (e.g., psychoanalytic, rational-emotive, or cognitive-behavioral), (c) therapeutic techniques (e.g., role playing, dream interpretation or positive regard), (d) homework assignments, and (e) any other interventions taking place inside or outside of the session.

TREATMENT PLAN FORMATS

Treatment plan formats vary, but at minimum, headings such as "Symptoms," "Goals/Objectives," and "Treatment Strategies" (or similar nomenclature) should be used. Some therapists include a separate column to list a time frame for attaining each objective. Others incorporate the same time period (e.g., 8 weeks, a particular date, or number of sessions) for the entire treatment plan, rather than setting separate time frames for reducing impairments. Some treatment plans include a column that lists specific services and providers to comply with JCAHO standards. Master treatment plans, such as those used in multidisciplinary settings, note which provider in the facility (and his or her area of specialty) will provide specific services and how often the services will be performed. When

TABLE 6.1
Methods for Measuring Behavioral Objectives

Type of measurement	Definition of objective	Sample statement of objective	Use
Time frames (Nominal data)	Objectives are identified by time periods in which behaviors will be evidenced/ decreased.	Client will remain sober for at least 30 days. Target date: July 9.	Easy to document by collaterals. Time is quantified, not the behavior.
Specific completion of assignments or tasks (Nominal data)	Documenting for med. evaluation, therapeutic contracts, homework, etc.	Client will visit psychiatrist by Dec. 12 for med. evaluation	Documents assignments given and additional services needed.
Specific outcomes (Nominal data)	Denoting whether or not behaviors have occurred.	Client will make no suicide attempts in next 60 days. Target date: February 12.	Generally objectives are rated by others. Used in day care or in residential settings.
Increase in frequency (Ordinal data)	Increases in positive behaviors	By May 8 the client will discuss in each group on average three incidents when he has not acted impulsively after getting his way.	Use when the goal is to increase frequency of behaviors.
Decrease in frequency (Ordinal data)	Decreases in negative target behaviors	The client will decrease suicidal threats to no more than 1/week by Dec. 12.	Use when the goal is to eliminate or decrease frequency of behaviors.
Baseline comparisons (Interval data)	Comparing levels of behaviors to a baseline measure	Client will increase positive statements to family. Current (baseline): 1/week Objective: 4/week by June 3.	Denoted in casenotes or graphs. Client easily visualizes progress as objectives are incrementally increased.

Note: Material adapted in collaboration with Steve Friedman, MA.

only one therapist provides services, as in private practice, no such notation is needed.

This text adopts the treatment plan format outlined in *The Complete Adult Psychotherapy Treatment Planner* (Jongsma & Peterson, 2003). This format complies with most third-party standards in which problem areas, goal, objectives, interventions, and diagnosis are listed.

COMMON PROBLEMS IN TREATMENT PLAN WRITING

If a therapist regards a treatment plan as an unnecessary document that is filled out simply because it is required by a third party, it will be of little or no benefit to the client because of the therapist's attitude toward having to fill out a perceived useless document. Without proper training as to the benefits of the treatment plan, therapists are likely to resist investing much energy into its formulation. Whether the writer has excellent or poor writing skills, they must be cognizant of its importance.

Treatment plan writing is vulnerable to several potential problems. The combination of documenting in a manner that complies with one or more regulatory agencies and third-party payer requirements, plus incorporating them into a brief document, requires creativity, writing skills, and knowledge of psychopathology and client-change agents.

Additional issues occur when the therapist lacks training regarding how to integrate diagnosis and treatment strategies, resulting in poorly documented treatment plans. Problems begin when the clinical assessment is unclear. Vague assessment procedures contribute to vague treatment plans, which lead to unfocused treatment. Other factors, such as developing nonmeasurable objectives and undefined treatment strategies, also lead to treatment with uncertain outcomes.

Problems also arise when the treatment plan does not correspond with the *DSM-IV-TR* diagnosis. Although treatment plans are not written for a diagnosis (they are written for client's specific strengths, needs, abilities, and preferences), they should reflect the diagnosis and resulting impairments. That is, a depressed client's treatment plan should address alleviated symptoms and impairment indicative of depression, not simply vague or global problem areas.

Therapeutic interventions listed in the treatment plan should not only be concordant with acceptable procedures in the mental health profession, but they should also be of proven effectiveness for the specific problems being treated. Generic treatment for all clients and problem areas is insufficient.

The number of goals and objectives should be consistent with the level of care and number of sessions allowed. Setting too many goals may overwhelm the client, and there may not be enough time to adequately address each goal in the allotted number of sessions. In addition, focusing too much on outcome measures may lead to treating symptoms rather than treating the client. On the other hand, underfocusing on outcomes promotes lack of therapeutic direction.

A well-written treatment plan is assessable. A reviewer should be able to read a treatment plan, then look at subsequent progress notes and treatment updates, and have a good idea of its effectiveness. Some common problems with treatment plans include the following:

- Vagueness
- Not indicative of the assessment
- Not incorporating both strengths and weakness
- Not addressing functional impairments
- Not reflecting the diagnosis
- Unrealistic (over- or underambitious)
- Not assessable

TREATMENT PLAN WRITING

The content of the treatment plan is based on information obtained in the diagnostic interview, psychological testing, collateral reports, observations, and previous treatment records. The treatment plan summarizes and prioritizes this information. Jongsma and Peterson (2003) suggest following these steps in developing the treatment plan.

STEP ONE: Problem Selection

Problem selection involves deciding which problem areas will be the focus of therapy. Although several problems may exist, they should be prioritized so that services will most effectively help the client. Problem areas should be expressed in behavioral terms. Remember that the treatment plan should list only problems that most effectively validate the diagnosis and show evidence of impairments.

STEP TWO: Problem Definition

The problems in step one should be defined according to the client's particular issues. Rather than resorting to generic definitions, problems should align with symptoms of a specific *DSM-IV-TR* or ISCD disorder and thereby correspond with a specific diagnosis. This specificity ensures that guidelines, such as JCAHO, are followed, and treatment is concordant with the diagnosis. Remember that problem areas should reflect areas of impairment in the client's life for which services are being sought. To ensure appropriate communication among mental health professionals, problems should be defined according to *DSM-IV-TR* terminology.

STEP THREE: Goal Development

Goals are broad descriptions of the desired outcome for each problem area. They specify behavior changes that the client must attain to demonstrate that treatment is working. Therapeutic techniques or strategies are used to reach goals but do not represent attainment of those goals. For example, the statement, "read two books about codependence," is not a goal because it does not suggest a behavior change; rather, it is a treatment strategy.

STEP FOUR: Objective Construction

Objectives are incremental steps to reaching goals. They must be observable and measurable to meet the requirements of third-party reviewers and fit a scientific-practitioner model. They directly correspond to the impairments (e.g., social, occupational, affective, physical) by which the diagnosis was validated. Generally, each goal should have at least two written objectives. Each objective should include a target date for attainment, at which time progress is evaluated and objectives are revised to more appropriately meet the underlying goals.

STEP FIVE: Intervention Creation

Interventions represent the treatment strategies conducted or guided by the therapist. Interventions should be empirically valid and not contraindicated or experimental. Each objective should have at least one intervention. Documentation of therapeutic interventions should include the type of therapy (e.g., individual, group, collateral, family), treatment modality (e.g.,psychodynamic, cognitive-behavioral, humanistic), and specific interventions common to the school of thought (e.g., role playing, dream interpretation, or bibliotherapy).

STEP SIX: Diagnosis Determination

The symptoms included in the treatment plan must be concordant with a *DSM-IV-TR* diagnosis. Few, if any, insurance companies will reimburse treatment without an Axis I diagnosis. Note that this author suggests that the diagnosis be determined prior to writing the treatment plan; however, step six is included to ensure that the treatment plan targets the client's diagnosis.

SAVING TIME IN WRITING TREATMENT PLANS

Both CARF and JCAHO (accrediting agencies) recommend that the client take an active part in establishing treatment plan goals and objectives. Some clinicians take time between sessions to write their treatment plans without consulting the client. A potential problem with this procedure is that it may leave out the client's SNAPs, and it could ignore important client needs.

Typically, the first session with the client is reserved for the diagnostic interview or assessment. The second session is dedicated to writing the treatment plan, in which the clinician and client can review the assessment material from the first session and cooperatively write the treatment plan together. This procedure increases client involvement in the treatment process and saves time. The session is usually quite therapeutic, providing clear client understanding of the direction for therapy and a better understanding by the therapist of the client's goals for treatment. The amount of time spent with the client in writing the treatment plan is affected by the client's level of motivation, insight, and cognitive functioning. It is advisable to spend less time and effort writing treatment plans in the session with clients with severe cognitive deficits, active psychotic concerns, or those with low motivation to be in treatment. In such cases clients typically need more direction from the therapist.

Example of dialog between a therapist (T) and a client (C) in collaborating in treatment plan writing:

T: In our initial meeting last week you mentioned a number of areas of change you would like to see in your life. Today we are going to work on writing your treatment plan, so we can plan what we will work on in therapy.

C: In the past I never had to help write the treatment plan. I just signed it and never saw it again. Can you just write one for me and start counseling?

T: That would be easy, but a treatment plan is designed to reflect what you want to accomplish in therapy. If we discuss your goals for therapy together, we are more likely to stay on target by treating specific problem areas that brought you to therapy. If not, it is very easy to go off in tangents in which therapy might take much longer than what is needed.

C: I see. It makes sense. So where do we start?

T: Well, we can first work on issues that are either most important, most stressful, or even less severe items if you want to ease yourself into the process of therapy.

C: What do you think I should do?

T: I can certainly help you with that decision, but I think it would mean more to you if we first looked at your ideas.

C: Okay. How about my panic attacks when I go outside? I'd like to learn to control them . . . and even have them eventually go away. Can we start there?

T: Sounds good. In the treatment plan we have terms called *goals* and *objectives*. Goals are the overall outcomes or results of therapy that you desire. Objectives are step-by-step means of reaching these goals. *(Therapist takes out a treatment plan form.)* Here, we have three columns, "Problem," "Goals/Objectives," and "Treatment Strategies." You mentioned that one of your problems is having panic attacks. Let's start there by writing "Panic Attacks" in the "Problem" column.

C: You're right. Panic attacks are a problem. *(Therapist writes "Panic Attacks" in the first column.)* So what do we put in the column marked "Goals/Objectives?"

T: Actually, you already answered part of the question. You said that you want to alleviate the panic attacks. Let's make that goal number one. *(Therapist writes, "Goal #1: Alleviate Panic Attacks" in column #2).*

C: So what about the objectives?

T: Good question. Let's look at our notes from last week. You said that panic attacks typically last about thirty minutes. Is that correct?

C: Yes, more or less, but thirty minutes is about average.

T: Objectives are specific behavioral improvements that you are trying to accomplish in a given time period. The goals are accomplished by gradually meeting various objectives that are increased each time they are reached. The final objective is to reach the goal. How would you like to set some objectives to be accomplished in the next four weeks? That doesn't mean that we'll be finished in four weeks, but it gives us more direction, and it brings us closer to the goal.

C: That sounds good. So what can we do in the next four weeks with my panic attacks?

T: Currently your panic attacks last for about thirty minutes. How about trying to cut down the time to under fifteen minutes by our session on September 30th? Does this seem reasonable to you?

C: Yes, it does. But what happens if I don't reach the objective or if I do much better?

T: Objectives are just estimates of what we believe can reasonably be accomplished. They can be revised periodically based on your progress.

C: It's good that there is room for not following the plan exactly.

T: How does this sound to you for goal 1, objective 1a? "Decrease duration of panic attacks from an average of thirty minutes to no more than fifteen minutes by September 30th." *(Therapist writes this as the 1a objective under Goal 1.)*

C: Yes, I would like that. It seems reachable, not too simple, not too difficult . . . I hope!"

T: Usually there are about three objectives for every goal. We do this to try to work on the problem by more than one means. You mentioned that panic attacks take place about three times per day. Perhaps we could have an objective to decrease the number of panic attacks per day.

C: Okay. How about going from three panic attacks per day to no more than one per day?

T: Alright. Under the first goal we'll write objective 1b, "Decrease frequency of panic attacks from an average of three per day to no more than one per day by September 30th." *(Therapist writes the objective under the objective 1a).*

C: What about a third objective?

T: It would be good to learn different means of relaxation when you feel panic symptoms emerging. How does that sound to you?

C: Could we make that objective 1c?

T: Yes, that would be fine. There are five relaxation techniques that I teach in therapy. It would be too much to teach them in one or two sessions. It is better to learn, practice, and master them one at a time to be most effective. I believe that it would be reasonable to learn two of them by September 30th. How does that sound to you?

C: I'm willing to learn and practice them if it helps.

T: We'll write objective 1c as, "Learn and implement two relaxation techniques to help prevent panic symptoms by September 30th. *(Therapist writes the objective under the objective 1b).*

C: What will we do to reach these goals and objectives?

T: The third column of the treatment plan is labeled "Treatment Strategies." It describes what we will be doing in therapy to attain the goals and objectives. This represents what we will do in and out of the counseling sessions.

C: What else is in the treatment plan?

T: Now, let's look at some other problems you mentioned last week and set up goals and objectives.

At this point the treatment plan looks like the one shown in Table 6.2.

TABLE 6.2
Sample Treatment Plan

Problem	Goals/Objectives	Treatment strategies
	(paraphrased from above narrative)	
1) Panic attacks occurring on an average of 3×/week for 30 minutes	Goal 1) Alleviate panic attacks	—Cognitive Therapy
	Obj 1a) Decrease duration to < 15 minutes by Sep. 30	—Teach relaxation
		—Med. referral
	Obj 1b) Decrease frequency to 0–1/day by Sep. 30	—Homework
		—Bibliotherapy
	Obj 1c) Learn 2 relaxation methods by Sep. 30	

REVISED TREATMENT PLANS

Treatment plans are not static documents. As treatment progresses, the objectives, treatment strategies, and circumstances change; thus, the treatment plan must reflect these modifications. There are three means of revising a treatment plan: *treatment plan revisions* and *revised treatment plans* and *treatment plan updates.*

Treatment plan revisions describe any changes that have taken place since the original treatment plan or previous update was written. The updates are typically written in the progress notes and might be listed in a treatment plan update form if one is used. For example, using the preceding treatment plan example, an update could be as simple as, "Revise Objective 1a to decrease duration of panic attacks to less than 8 minutes." If the goal for a problem area has been met, it could be written as, "Goal 1, Alleviate panic attacks met." Or, if additional problem areas and goals are set, they would be added to the treatment plan.

A *revised treatment plan* is a rewritten treatment plan reflecting current progress. It generally includes a brief narrative of progress to date. Objectives that have been met are revised to more closely reflect goals. Those that have not been met are reviewed to determine if other interventions could be more helpful. New objectives may also be introduced into the treatment plan at this point. A revised treatment plan, then, is similar to the original treatment plan, but it reflects the client's current state of functioning. Most of the information has been taken from the periodic treatment plan revisions. It is common to revise a treatment plan every 60 to 90 days. As in the initial treatment plan, it is formulated collaboratively by the client and therapist.

A *treatment plan update* is similar or identical to a preauthorization for additional services report, which will be explained in Chapter 8. A sample request for additional services is found on page 192. Overall, the update is a summary of how treatment plan objectives have been met to date, providing evidence of the effectiveness of the therapeutic interventions.

A properly documented treatment plan provides a solid foundation for documenting the course of therapy. Once the treatment plan has been developed, the next step is to put the plan into action. To keep therapy time-efficient and on track and to qualify for reimbursement, clinicians must document that the plan is being followed and progress is being made. Progress notes serve this purpose.

Progress notes are the only documentation that shows third-party reviewers the degree to which treatment is effective. Chapter 7 demonstrates how to write effective progress notes that are concordant with the treatment plan.

HIGHLIGHTS
of Chapter 6

★ Although a relatively new procedure, the treatment plan is the most frequently consulted treatment document.

★ There is a major difference between planning treatment and writing a treatment plan.

★ Because a diagnosis is based on the *DSM-IV-TR*, the treatment plan also validates *DSM-IV-TR* principles.

★ Treatment plans are designed to provide observable and measurable treatment outcome measures that demonstrate alleviation of functional impairments.

★ Both the client and therapist take an active part in treatment plan formulation.

★ Treatment plans are highly individualized and account for several client and therapist variables, situational concerns, and third-party regulations.

★ The client ultimately sets the goals and objectives for treatment.

★ Goals reflect overall outcomes in therapy, whereas objectives are incremental, objective, and measurable steps by which goals are attained.

★ Objectives are periodically revised as treatment progresses toward the goals.

★ There are several ways to measure objectives, which allows for variations in techniques and schools of thought.

QUESTIONS

1. Which of the following best represents a treatment plan *objective?*

 (a) Eliminate depression

 (b) Return to work at least 30 hours per week

 (c) Initiate cognitive therapy

 (d) Prozac, 40 mg

2. Which of the following best represents a treatment plan *goal?*

 (a) Return to work full time

 (b) Begin psychoanalysis

 (c) Visit physician for evaluation

 (d) Enter group therapy for 12 weeks

3. Which of the following provides the best example of a measurable behavioral objective?

 (a) Continue therapy

 (b) Increase sense of well being

 (c) Discuss previous treatment

 (d) Spend at least 3 hours per week outdoors

4. What is wrong with the following treatment plan objective? Objective: Increase euthymic mood.

 (a) It is too vague.

 (b) It is difficult to measure.

 (c) Both of these.

 (d) Nothing. It is a good objective.

5. The treatment plan is primarily designed to be based on

 (a) specific client needs.

 (b) the diagnosis.

 (c) the therapist's specialty.

 (d) the therapist's theoretical school of thought.

6. Any treatment plan revisions are typically written

    (a) in the form of a new treatment plan.

    (b) in homework assignments by the client.

    (c) in the initial diagnostic interview and accomplished gradually throughout treatment.

    (d) in the progress notes, then incorporated into the revised treatment plan.

Answers: 1. b; 2. a; 3. d; 4. c; 5. a; 6. d

7

Progress Notes

Progress notes provide evidence, not only that a session took place, but also of the effects of treatment. They are the only record for documenting the session's length, type, content, interventions, and therapeutic progress. Because progress notes are the primary source for documenting what happens in therapy and the level of progress is being made, they are a primary document reviewed by auditors. Clinicians must be certain, therefore, that session content is not simply implied but rather fully documented.

A reader should be able to ascertain the client's diagnosis, current issues, and effects of therapy from reading progress notes. Progress notes correspond with the client's presenting problems and the diagnosis. It is also necessary to document a client's functional impairments that have led to the medical necessity for services, plus the course of treatment toward alleviating those impairments. For example, if a client is diagnosed with depression, the progress notes should primarily reflect treatment for depression and not other areas (unless they, too, have been included in the treatment plan). That is, areas treated must be in the treatment plan.

Progress notes have evolved with increasing importance over the years. Older methods merely documented that a session was held and informed the reader to some degree of what happened in the session. Today, progress notes are an essential documentation tool. Third-party criteria for progress notes have become progressively more stringent in terms of accountability because traditionally there has been little documented evidence of the effects of therapy. Requirements for demonstrating outcomes in mental health treatment are increasing (Wiger & Solberg, 2001).

Third-party requirements, whether they are from regulatory agencies or third-party payers, demand behavioral evidence to demonstrate accountability for services. For financial reasons, third-party payers cannot provide unlimited mental health benefits. Regulatory agencies set high standards to raise the level of accountability and professionalism in the mental health field. Therapists must clearly document that the treatment plan is being followed and services are being directed toward the active symptoms of the diagnosis, what progress is being made, and how goals and objectives are being addressed.

Why Write Progress Notes?

In addition to third-party requirements regarding the use of progress notes, there are other benefits as well. Progress notes establish accountability to the client. Keeping therapy on track and steadily noting progress by following the treatment plan assures cost-effectiveness. Progress notes are designed to provide evidence that the services being conducted are efficacious.

It is unlikely that, over any length of time, a therapist can remember the specific points and interventions in every session. When reviewing a client's chart prior to a session, therapists can refresh their memories as to the client's ongoing concerns, treatments employed, homework assignments, and progress toward treatment plan goals. A therapist who does not remember the content of previous sessions is likely to be viewed in a different light by a client than a therapist who is up to date with the records.

Well-kept progress notes may help protect the therapist from litigious or ethical problems that might arise without adequate documentation. For example, in the beginning of this writer's career as a psychologist, a client had attempted suicide the day after an intake session. Immediately, this psychologist was contacted by the client's family interrogating as to how this potential problem wasn't discovered during the intake interview. The notes indicated that a number of questions regarding suicide were posed, but the client denied that there were such concerns. The suicide attempt was a reaction to a crisis that had taken place the day after the evaluation. Although suicide is extremely difficult to predict (Wiger & Harowski, 2003; Maltsberger, 1988; Hillard, 1995), the therapist must carefully document observations and client statements regarding such issues.

Progress notes are also helpful when a client is transferred to another therapist. Clear progress notes alert the new therapist regarding specific issues that have been addressed and the types of interventions that work best for the client. Without sufficient records of treatment, the client would basically have to start over when changing therapists, leading to unnecessary, wasted time at the client's expense. Transitioning from one therapist to another is enough of an ordeal for a client, which shouldn't be exacerbated by poor communication between the therapists involved.

Progress notes also establish baseline behaviors to help evaluate progress and setbacks. Perhaps one of the best means of evaluating the outcomes of treatment is a review of the data documented in the progress notes. Notations such as compliance, attendance, insight, alleviation of impairments, cyclical behaviors, and much more provide helpful information to best serve the client.

The HIPAA regulations have changed the availability of progress notes to someone requesting a client's health records. Historically, when a client's medical information was requested, it was common to copy the entire file. The HIPAA requires that the minimum necessary information be sent to someone requesting medical records. In addition, progress notes are to be kept separate from the client's main file. Progress notes may be sent when asked for specifically, with the client's (or designated representative's) permission.

WHAT CONSTITUTES A GOOD PROGRESS NOTE?

Although not every progress note from every session covers each of these topics, overall they should address the following questions:

1. What content or topics were discussed in the session?
2. How did the session address treatment plan objectives?
3. What therapeutic interventions and techniques were employed and how effective were they?
4. What clinical observations (behavioral, affective, etc.) were made?
5. What progress or setbacks occurred?
6. What signs and symptoms of the diagnosis are present, increasing, decreasing, or no longer present?

7. How are the treatment plan goals and objectives being met at this time?

8. What is the current medical necessity for services?

9. What is being done outside the session?

10. What are the client's current limitations and strengths?

Answering these questions documents that appropriate treatment is being provided. It is not necessary to address each question in every progress note; rather, a pattern of documentation should be established so that each question is adequately addressed over the course of therapy. Let's consider each question individually.

What Content or Topics Were Discussed in the Session?

Historically, progress notes have provided a summary of what took place in the session. Although this information is important, it does not necessarily document medical necessity. Statements should be objective and factual, including information regarding current, on-going, or historical events in the client's life. In addition, validation of the diagnosis and evidence that the treatment plan is being followed are important aspects of progress notes. Documenting session content is necessary but not sufficient if nothing else is written in the progress notes.

Contentwise, progress notes should include the main topics discussed in the session. If more than one topic is discussed, each topic should be listed in the order it was addressed. Topic areas should coincide with the areas of strength and weakness addressed in the treatment plan. If topic areas do not seem to relate to the primary purpose of treatment, the purpose and medical necessity for covering the topic should be documented, and, if continued to additional sessions, it should be added to treatment plan revisions.

Examples of content-oriented progress note statements include the following:

- "Discussed ways in which family of origin influences current behaviors."
- "Session focused on the four times client has been in the hospital for suicidal gestures."
- "Client asked to help explore problems coping with rejection."

How Did the Session Address Treatment Plan Objectives?

As noted, one of the main functions of progress notes is to document that treatment plan goals and objectives are being addressed. Progress notes should specify which treatment plan objectives are being treated and how they are progressing.

If, for example, a treatment plan addresses the client's depressed mood in each problem area, goal, and objective, but progress notes document that communication skills in the client's marriage are the focus of treatment, treatment plan goals and objectives are not being addressed or met. To avoid this, it is helpful to assign a number or letter to each treatment goal and objective and list in the progress notes which ones are being treated in each session. It is common to denote the goal as a number and the related objectives as alphabetical characters following the number. For example:

Goal 1: Increase self-esteem.

Objective 1a: Initiate at least 2 positive behaviors per week, as identified in Session 2.

Objective 1b: Employ at least 3 assertive behaviors per week.

In this case, the progress note statement could read: "Worked on Objective 1b by role playing various assertive behaviors." Additional statements could indicate specific issues and interventions being employed to address treatment objectives.

What Therapeutic Interventions and Techniques Were Employed and How Effective Were They?

Progress notes include describing the specific therapeutic interventions taking place during the session. Some treatment strategies are more effective than others, depending on the diagnosis and client variables. In addition, some treatment strategies are experimental, and others have been demonstrated to be nonefficacious in certain therapeutic situations. It is not unusual for a third-party insurance or managed care contract to specifically state that the policy does not cover experimental therapeutic procedures.

The treatment plan lists which therapeutic school of thought and procedures will be employed in the treatment. Progress notes verify that the procedures are being used and demonstrate the outcomes of implementing the procedures. Such documentation helps the clinician evaluate the effectiveness of treatment and decide whether changes to the treatment plan should be made.

Documenting specific treatment interventions also helps the therapist keep the session on track and therapeutic. Without them, sessions could deteriorate to chit-chat or discussions irrelevant to treatment. Examples include the following:

- "Utilized empty chair technique to help client find closure from divorce. Client wept through the entire procedure, later stating that he felt better because he had been holding in too many feelings."

- "Client states that she does not want to practice relaxation techniques in the sessions anymore because they make her more upset."

What Clinical Observations (Behavioral, Affective, etc.) Were Made?

The therapist's clinical observations are crucial in evaluating both the course of therapy and assessing the client's current condition. Notations should include clinically significant observations of verbal and nonverbal behaviors. Observations should be integrated with the client's presenting problem and diagnostic concerns. For example, if a client is diagnosed with depression, progress notes should regularly assess the client's level of depression. It is expected that the client would appear less depressed as therapy progresses. Unless progress notes document these observations, there is no way to assess the efficacy of treatment.

Examples of clinical observations include the following:

- "The client appeared depressed as evidenced by slumped posture, crying often, and a blunted affect."

- "The client appeared anxious as evidenced by speaking more rapidly than usual, hyperventilating, sweating, and getting out of the chair four times."

- "The child continues to demonstrate defiant behaviors as evidenced by yelling at her mother three times during the session, telling this therapist to "stuff it," and refusing to answer questions over 50% of the time."

Each of these progress note statements documents observations that validate the diagnosis and treatment plan. Without statements of this nature, a third-party auditor or insurance case manager may not find sufficient evidence to warrant payment for additional services. There have been legal and ethics cases in which treatment is rendered to a client, but the progress notes did not clearly document that a disorder existed or was properly treated. Results have led to licensure issues, malpractice, or other disciplinary measures. Concise documentation helps solve all of these issues.

What Progress or Setbacks Occurred?

Because behavioral health insurers routinely rely on a scientific model to substantiate treatment and a significant number of clients utilize such insurance to pay for treatment, it is necessary that this model be used to document a client's impairments and the medical necessity for treatment. In this model, treatment that does not alleviate or reduce impairments is not considered helpful and should be discontinued or modified.

> Consider a person with a broken leg who visited the doctor at regular intervals for treatment. It would be expected that the patient's medical charts would document the specific medical procedures and service, plus the timely improvements in the patient's condition. When the patient returned to normal functioning and the leg was healed, the appointments would end. If the broken bone began to deteriorate, we would expect it to be clearly documented to help determine necessary changes in the treatment. Mental health services documentation follows a similar method.

Third-party payers will generally stop reimbursing treatment that does not document alleviation of impairments after a number of sessions or after various interventions have been attempted without positive results. There are a number of possible reasons why a client might not improve, or even decompensate, in therapy. In such cases the therapist should document each attempt to revise the client's treatment (e.g., new strategies, increased number of sessions, additional services, change in environment, medications, change therapists, other referrals). When no progress takes place, despite the increased efforts, decisions must be made regarding future treatment. At some point, though, the possibility of discontinued payment becomes a concern.

Conversely, it is also possible for a client to progress in leaps and bounds due to excellent treatment, but not qualify for reimbursement because progress notes were poorly written. In such cases, the therapist is advised to seek supervision in documentation procedures because both the client and the therapist suffer. Too many promising therapists have become discouraged or left the field due to factors other than their counseling ability. These "other factors" can be learned.

Clinical setbacks do not necessarily indicate that treatment is of poor quality. Setbacks might occur because additional stressors develop during the course of therapy, treatment strategies are not the best fit for the client, the client-therapist match is not optimum, the client is noncompliant, or for a number of other reasons. Documenting setbacks is important because it raises red flags indicating that changes are likely needed. Good documentation explains how clinical setbacks were handled and how subsequent changes affected the client's condition.

Clear documentation of progress and setbacks makes it easier for the clinician to consult with other professionals about the case. Examples of progress note statements of progress and setbacks include the following:

- "Progress is evidenced by client's initiating discussions in session, displaying a normal affect, and no longer crying during session when discussing losing his job."

- "The client states that she has been more depressed and frustrated in the past three weeks because her family is protesting her attempts to be more assertive."

- "The child's mother states that target behaviors in school (hitting teacher, stealing, and destroying property) have escalated to the point of being suspended from school."

What Signs and Symptoms of the Diagnosis Are Present or No Longer Present?

The medical model requires documenting the presence or absence of symptoms and impairments reflective of the need for services.

Just as a diagnosis is validated by the presence of symptoms and impairments, progress is assessed by alleviation of symptoms and impairments. In effect, the initial diagnostic interview identifies symptoms and impairments, and treatment attempts to resolve or alleviate them. Most psychotherapies do not actively or specifically focus on symptoms alone as part of the therapeutic process. Symptoms and impairment reduction is a documentation procedure, not necessarily a therapeutic technique.

There is a notable difference between a medical model of therapy and a medical model of documentation. A medical model of documentation can be used for any type of therapy, whether the treatment focuses on symptoms, insight, the relationship, cognitions, behavior, or anything else. No matter what theoretical model is practiced, the client will have some sort of gauge of the level of therapeutic progress. For example, if a client who previously experienced an average of three panic attacks per day prior to therapy now reports having one or none per day, symptoms have been reduced. The client's primary concern is not the type of treatment used; what is important is the decrease in panic attacks. Thus, although the medical model is used to document the effects of therapy, it is not needed to determine the process or method used in treatment.

Clients have a reason for coming to therapy. Generally, something in their lives is not going well. Issues might be related to emotional, social, occupational, or other aspects of their lives. The reason a client comes to therapy is called the *presenting problem*. If clients are able to detect that they need services due to subjective levels of symptoms and impairments, they will also know when they are getting better. Effective progress notes document these changes in client symptoms and impairments. For example:

- "The client claims to be symptom-free of binging and purging for the past two months."

- "Since the onset of therapy, the client claims to feel increasingly more irritable."

- "The client states that she is no longer depressed most of the time. Previously she endorsed feeling depressed at least six days per week. Currently she states that she feels depressed no more than one to two days per week."

How Are Treatment Plan Goals and Objectives Being Met at This Time?

Progress notes regularly evaluate the effectiveness of therapy. Measurable and observable treatment plan objectives provide the best evidence of therapeutic effectiveness. Progress note statements may be evaluative or summative, or they may provide current information about the client's progress. Statements of this nature are helpful in making treatment plan revisions. For example:

- "Four out of five treatment goals have been met to date. Client states that he is feeling much better and is considering discharge in the next two weeks."

- Objective 2b, "attend work at least three days per week," is met and being revised to "attend work at least four days per week."

- "Little progress has been made in the past two months of treatment, due to noncompliance."

- "Considerable setbacks are noted in Objective 3b in which the homework assignments appear to be too stressful for the client. The client appears to be more anxious socially since given the assignment of greeting three neighbors per day. The treatment strategies for this objective will be changed to bibliotherapy and role playing at this time."

What Is the Current Medical Necessity for Services?

Most insurers require evidence of medical necessity as a requirement for reimbursing mental health services. Thus, progress notes should document the medical necessity of services needed by regularly recording the client's functional impairments caused by the mental illness.

According to a medical model, when a client is no longer functionally impaired, services are no longer necessary. Documentation of functional behaviors thus helps the therapist and client to decide when treatment can be terminated. When treatment plan goals, objectives, and discharge criteria are written clearly and understood by both the client and the therapist, vagary about termination decreases.

On the other hand, some therapy is not considered medically necessary by third-party payers, including counseling solely for personal growth, psychoeducational treatment, treatment for non-Axis I disorders, and other types of therapy in which the client is not significantly impaired by a mental disorder. Although clinicians need not necessarily steer clear from those types of therapy, they may have to prepare patients to be prepared to pay the bill themselves. Unfortunately, some third-party payers forbid their contracted therapists from charging for mental health services that are not medically necessary. Some examples of documenting continued medical necessity include the following:

- "The client has experienced an average of five panic attacks daily, lasting twenty to thirty minutes, leading to going home from work early most days or missing work most days."

- "Since the onset of medication and insight-oriented therapy, the client has been able to get out of bed at least three days per week but remains unable to go to classes."

- "Discussed termination of services due to significant progress in meeting therapeutic goals, which has led to a return to normal functioning socially and occupationally."

What Is Being Done Outside the Session to Increase Effectiveness of Therapy?

Although most psychotherapy occurs at the clinician's office, progress is not measured solely in the context of isolated in-office sessions. Although the clinician can observe progress in session, most indices of progress are statements reported by the client or collaterals about behaviors that occur outside the session. Thus, it is important to document these statements as well. Such documentation may include compliance and progress of homework assignments, behaviors generalized from the sessions, and interventions utilizing collaterals. For example:

- "Client reports initiating three conversations at school party, as rehearsed in the previous session. Reports decreased anxiety resulting from rehearsal."

- "Client's spouse reports enhanced marital satisfaction due to increased positive remarks made since onset of marital therapy."

- "Compliance in homework assignments remains at over 80%."

What Are the Client's Current Limitations and Strengths?

Throughout the course of therapy, a client's limitations and strengths will change. Strengths will increase due to compliance with effective therapy. But as the effects of therapy impact the client's family and other environmental systems, certain stressors will also increase. Behavioral changes in one family member are most likely to disrupt the family system in one way or another.

Even the most dysfunctional client possesses strengths that can be incorporated into the treatment process. Client strengths should be assessed throughout the therapeutic process and incorporated into treatment even though weaknesses and impairments often seem to be the focus of therapy in a medical model. For example, if a person injures his or her right arm, use of the left arm is apt to increase because it is a strength. As the right arm heals, there will be less reliance on the left arm. If only the left or right arm receive attention, the healing process will be hampered, due to over- or underuse. Documenting client strengths and stressors could include statements such as the following:

- "The client continues utilizing social supports, such as family and friends, when feeling an urge to consume alcohol."
- "The client is improving in reducing levels of anxiety by utilizing relaxation techniques employed in therapy."
- "Although the client is learning new coping mechanisms, his family is refusing to trust him to be alone by himself. Much frustration is reported."
- "The client describes feeling much better and more comfortable around others since volunteering at the youth center using his carpentry skills."

OTHER ITEMS ADDRESSED IN PROGRESS NOTES

In addition to the items discussed previously, progress notes should include other important information, such as the following:

1. *Type of sessions being conducted (e.g., individual, family, group).* Progress notes should list specific types of therapy and therapeutic techniques and describe their effectiveness. Some auditors validate the type of therapy via progress notes. For example, if a therapist bills an insurance company for individual psychotherapy but progress notes document marital therapy, reimbursement may be denied. (Few insurance companies pay for marital counseling.) Billing marital counseling as individual or family counseling is considered insurance fraud.

2. *Goals and objectives addressed in the session.* Third-party payers provide guidelines such as, "Progress notes must reflect the objectives of the treatment plan." Some progress note forms allow space to list the treatment plan objectives being addressed in the session. Even if the form does not have space for this, clinicians should consider listing session objectives to keep sessions on target.

3. *Time frame of the session: date, starting time, ending time, duration.* Each progress note should list the time frame of the session. This author recalls an audit in which the evaluator complained that noting the length of a session as "one hour" was not sufficient, stating, "How do I know the session lasted one hour unless you write down both the starting and ending times?"

4. *Signature and credentials of the therapist (initials only are insufficient).* After the session, the therapist should sign the progress note with his or her full signature, including professional credentials (degree and licensure), which denotes professional responsibility for the session. Initials are not sufficient for such an endorsement just as a check cannot be cashed without a valid signature.

Poorly Written Progress Notes versus Well-Written Progress Notes

Figure 7.1 illustrates the difference between a poorly documented progress note and a properly documented one. The following dialogue between a client and his therapist provides background for the documentation:

C: I'm so upset about everything that has been happening to me.
T: Tell me what you mean.
C: Ever since I was fired from my job everyone is out to get me.
T: Everyone?
C: Yes. My ex-boss at work won't pay for unemployment compensation. My wife thinks I'm a bum. The police are following me. My food tastes funny, if you know what I mean. My children don't want to play with me. Yes, everyone is out to get me.

FIGURE 7.1
Progress Note Statements

Poorly Written Progress Note

We talked about issues at home and on the job. Increased fears and marriage problems. Spouse is cheating on him. Not communicating well. Complaining about spouse, job, and police.

The progress note does not depict the medical necessity of services. Although the content might be accurate, it is unclear diagnostically, symptomatically, therapeutically, and it does not depict current impairments. Even though significant impairments may exist, the evidence provided is so poor an auditor would most likely state that there is lack of justification to continue services. Statements such as "spouse is cheating on him," may or may not be accurate, therefore should be written as a belief, quote, or not at all. None of the questions listed on pages 145–146 were addressed.

Properly Documented Progress Note

Client appeared nervous, tense, and guarded, noting several current stressors. Was easily upset and agitated when discussing ongoing issues. Recently fired from job. Much blaming of others (ex-employer, spouse, police) of following him, spying on him, being unfaithful to him or trying to harm him. Often got up and looked out of the window for police. Confirms having a longstanding history of not trusting others

---

Although progress note remarks are brief, they more clearly indicate current impairments, validate diagnostic criteria, and demonstrate the need for further services. The progress note briefly discussed a possible antecedent (recently fired from his job), resulting exacerbation of nontrusting behaviors (increased paranoia with ex-employer, spouse, and police), and impairments (distrust, checking behaviors, affective concerns).

T: How long have you believed that people are out to get you?

C: Well, I've never trusted anyone completely (speaking more rapidly), but I knew for sure a few months ago when my boss warned me that people at work were complaining about my so-called attitude, as she puts it. I told her what I thought about the situation, and they fired me. (In a much louder voice) I knew it would happen.

T: What about the police following you?

C: Oh, yes. Yesterday I noticed police driving by the house at least four times (carefully looks out the window). They were acting like they weren't looking for me, but I know their tactics. I'm sure they're bugging my phone. Have they talked to you about me?

T: And the food tasting funny?

C: My wife does all of the cooking. There's something different in the taste the past few months. I'm sure she's in on it, too. Who knows who she's sleeping with now.

T: Now?

C: Yes, we've been married only one year . . . it's my second mar-riage . . . I've always wondered why she doesn't answer the phone when I call her in the afternoon. Come on, let's get real (sarcastically). We all can add two plus two. I won't get near her or any of my so-called friends. Just leave me alone.

SCIENTIFIC METHOD

According to the scientific method, measurements are based on a baseline behavior, and subsequent measures determine a client's degree of change. Without a baseline measure, the level of change is difficult to assess. Baselines may be established in the diagnostic interview and throughout therapy, and progress note documenta-tion can incorporate changes to the baselines. Two documentation methods utilizing the scientific model are commonly used.

Comparative

In this case, the clinician documents various baseline measures that depict current impairments. These measures may be docu-mented in the intake notes, psychological report, treatment plan, or in progress notes. A progress note might report, "Since the onset of Ritalin (15 mg. $\times$ 2) the client's teacher reports the client being on task 80% of the time, compared to 50% prior to treatment."

Behavioral Charts

With this method, either the therapist, client, or collaterals chart progress throughout therapy. Progress notes generally refer to the client's chart to register progress or setbacks. An excellent use of charting to document therapeutic progress incorporates treatment plan goals and objectives throughout therapy. Figure 7.2 illustrates how one picture is worth a thousand words.

FIGURE 7.2
Charting Client Progress over Course of Therapy

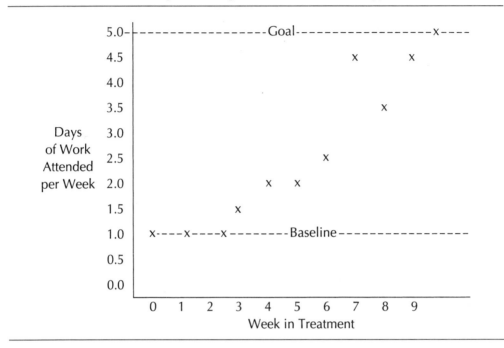

PROGRESS NOTE FORMATS

Clinicians use several formats or means of organizing progress notes. The most popular formats are SOAP and DAP. SOAP (Subjective, Objective, Assessment, Plan) progress notes contain four sections, whereas DAP (Data, Assessment, Plan) progress notes include three categories.

SOAP	DAP
Subjective	**D**ata
Objective	**A**ssessment
Assessment	**P**lan
Plan	

The Assessment and Plan portions of both DAP and SOAP notes are identical. The only difference between SOAP and DAP progress notes is how session content is organized. A DAP progress note lists session content as Data, whereas SOAP progress notes break down session content data into two types: Subjective and Objective.

Data

SOAP Progress Notes

The subjective data of SOAP notes are not quantifiable or measurable; rather, they include subjective statements reflecting the client's condition. Information includes the client's presenting problems and historical data (e.g., family background, medical history, and social structure). Examples of subjective data include the following:

- "The client reports feeling sad most of the time."
- "He states that he is from a dysfunctional family."
- "Several physical concerns were reported such as . . ."

The objective section of SOAP notes represents observable data. Objective data provide specific information that can be compared to previous data or used as a baseline for future objective observations. Examples of objective data include the following:

- "Current score on the Beck Depression Inventory was 13, which is significantly lower than 28, recorded two months ago."
- "She appeared dysphoric the entire session."
- "On three occasions he cried, stating that he wants to give up trying."

DAP Progress Notes

The DAP format is becoming more popular and is considered by many to be more user-friendly than the SOAP format. For this reason, this book will utilize the DAP format. For DAP progress notes, the therapist does not have to separate two types of data (subjective and objective) into different portions of the progress note. Also, some statements, such as "The patient appeared confused, as evidenced by rambling 50% of the session," contain both subjective and objective information that is difficult to separate in the progress notes.

Assessment

The assessment section of the progress note (the same for SOAP and DAP formats) is a written evaluation of the current session and how it relates to the cumulative scope of therapy. The following are types of information documented in this section:

1. Effects or results of the current session
2. Therapeutic progress
3. Client's level of cooperation/insight/motivation
4. Client progress and setbacks
5. Areas requiring more clinical work
6. Effectiveness of treatment strategies
7. Completion of treatment plan objectives
8. Changes needed to keep therapy on target
9. Need for diagnostic revisions

Although it is not necessary to address each area in every progress note, each should be covered sufficiently over the course of therapy. The statements in the Assessment section are summaries of the information in the Data section. Consider each item individually:

1. *Effects of the Current Session*   Comments assessing the effectiveness of the session are limited to data collected during the specific session. These comments are not meant to assess the cumulative effects of the course of treatment. For example:

- "The session seemed helpful in eliciting the client's feelings about how he resents his family intruding on his marriage."
- "The session was not helpful in building rapport."

2. *Therapeutic Progress*   Statements assessing the course of therapy document the overall effects of therapeutic interventions rather than the effects of the current session. Third-party reviewers regularly request this information. When progress notes consistently document the course of therapy, the clinician does not have to search for this information because it will be located in the assessment portion of each progress note. For example:

- "The client continues to show steady progress in therapy."
- "Group therapy has not been beneficial to this point."

3. *Client's Level of Cooperation/Insight/Motivation*   Client variables require the clinician's careful attention. An excellent therapist will be ineffective without mutual cooperation. The client's level of motivation and insight should be assessed to help evaluate whether the current regimen of treatment is sufficient. For example:

- "The client appears to have adequate insight into the nature of his therapeutic issues."
- "Level of cooperation has increased in the past month, leading to increased compliance in homework assignments and behavioral changes."

4. *Client Progress and Setbacks*   It is crucial to document both progress and setbacks. Such documentation provides regular assessments of what positive and negative outcomes have occurred since the onset of treatment. If only progresses are documented, it appears that there is no need for continued services. If only setbacks are documented, it appears that therapy is not helping.

- "The client has increased suicidal threats, posing an increased risk to herself."
- "Significant client progress is noted in reducing anxiety and worrying."

5. *Areas Requiring More Clinical Work*   Throughout therapy, clients will experience ongoing changes and stressors in their lives. New issues will surface, and others will be alleviated. As the client progresses through therapy, new stressors will develop due to behavioral and environmental changes resulting from therapy. For example, if a client is taught to be more assertive, it may impact the dynamics of the client's family, thereby raising new therapeutic issues. Certain issues that may have been considered minor in the original assessment may develop into significant problem areas. Impairments apparent at the time of the initial assessment might have only a marginal impact upon the client's current functioning level. Current documentation of medical necessity is based on client impairments; therefore, impairments should be assessed periodically to help determine the current need for services. The original treatment plan may suffice for a certain period of time, but eventually the clinical direction will need to be revised. The assessment section allows clinicians to note changes in the client's life that may require revising the treatment plan. For example:

- "Slight progress has taken place in alleviating temper tantrums, but school reports indicate continued need to focus on his bullying behavior."
- "The client's excessive drinking of alcohol and not looking for a job continue to cause severe financial and family problems that attribute to client's anxiety and depression."
- "The client no longer reports having panic attacks prior to meeting new people."

6. *Effectiveness of Treatment Strategies*   Treatment strategies should also be assessed periodically. Strategies that are particularly effective or ineffective should be noted and, if necessary, revised. Documenting whether treatment strategies work benefits future treatment providers who work with the client. For example:

- "Most progress has occurred when the client is given a homework assignment that corresponds to the session topic."
- "Client seems to lack insight, but behavioral strategies are effective in meeting treatment plan goals."

7. *Completion of Treatment Plan Objectives*   Third-party payers require periodic updates to the treatment plan. The underlying question focuses on whether the goals and objectives are being met. If they are not being met, or if progress is slower than expected, services may not be considered cost effective. Thus, other services may be more efficacious for the client and should be considered. For example:

- "Treatment plan objectives 2a, 3b, and 4a have been accomplished."
- "Client has not been able to return to college by the target date, due to excessive social anxiety."

8. *Changes Needed to Keep Therapy on Target*   Therapy is a dynamic process. Problem areas and objectives change on a regular basis. Every setback and achievement sets new directions, no matter how slight. Assessment of needed changes provides a periodic look at the direction therapy is heading and what overall changes will most benefit the client. For example:

- "The client is under significant stress at this time, and monthly psychotherapy is not sufficient to meet her therapeutic needs."
- "The client seems to be uncomfortable disclosing personal information to a male therapist. This therapist suggests referral to a female therapist."

9. *Need for Diagnostic Revisions* As more information is gathered about the client and life stressors change, the clinician may revise a diagnosis based on recent information. Some disorders go into remission, whereas others no longer fit *DSM-IV-TR* time frames. The specific reasons for changing a diagnosis should be listed in the Data (DAP format) section, but the overall assessment of the client should be listed in the Assessment section. Some clinicians periodically assess the current diagnosis by validating current symptoms and restating the diagnosis in the Assessment section. For example:

- "Based on additional information, the diagnosis of Oppositional Defiant Disorder will be revised to Conduct Disorder."
- "The client continues meeting criteria for Bipolar II Disorder."

Plan

The Plan section of progress notes is also identical for SOAP and DAP formats. Just as the Assessment is based on the Data (subjective and objective types for SOAP notes), the Plan is based on the Assessment. The Plan section of the progress notes documents the focus of future treatment based on the client's current functioning level. Noting future plans for therapy also helps the therapist keep track of treatment options and follow up on assignments. It includes plans for use inside and outside of the session, such as the following:

1. Homework assignments
2. Upcoming interventions

3. Content of future sessions

4. Treatment plan revisions

5. Referrals

Homework Assignments

Homework assignments include any assigned tasks to be completed outside of the counseling session. They range from behavioral assignments, to charting progress, to reading to meditating. Homework should relate to the treatment plan and be designed to increase functioning. When homework is assigned, it is important to write it down in the Plan section, so the therapist can review it prior to the next session and be prepared to discuss it at the next session. For example:

- "The client will write a letter to his parents describing his thoughts and feelings about how they treat his sister better than him."
- "Continue logging feelings of anger."
- "Loaned client a copy of *I'm OK, You're OK* to discuss next week."

Upcoming Interventions

There are times when a therapist decides to try a new treatment strategy in a future session. When planning future session topics or interventions, it is helpful to discuss them in advance with the client. For example:

- "Next session: Incorporate role playing of assertiveness with best friend."
- "Incorporate systematic desensitization during the next several sessions."

Content of Future Sessions

Treatment plans generally list at least two or three problem areas that will be addressed during the course of therapy. It is possible to dwell on one problem area for the duration of treatment and never address other areas of the treatment plan. To avoid this, it is helpful to plan in advance when some or all of the client's problems will be discussed and then periodically review the treatment plan with the client to ensure that problem areas are being adequately addressed. For example:

- "Next session: Treatment plan problem area #2, binge eating."
- "Continue treatment of self-esteem issues."

Treatment Plan Revisions

Treatment plans are designed to be revised when client impairments change. This does not mean that the treatment plan must be rewritten each time any progress or setbacks occur. As objectives are met (or not met), they should be revised in an effort to meet treatment goals. New treatment strategies may be added as more information about the client is learned. For example:

- "Current objective: Maximum of five panic attacks daily. Revised objective: Maximum of two panic attacks daily."
- "New objective: Apply for a minimum of three employment positions per week."

Referrals

Any referrals or additional services suggested that affect current treatment should also be documented in the Plan section. For example:

- "Referred to Dr. Smith for medical evaluation."
- "Referred client to Alcoholics Anonymous."

Third-party payers will often ask if a medical or psychiatric referral was given, so it is important to note referrals in the client's chart. The Data section of future progress notes will document the effects of client compliance with the referral. Figure 7.3 provides a DAP progress note for John Doe.

John Doe's progress note follows specific treatment plan objectives and interventions. It validates continued medical necessity by providing examples of current symptoms and impairments concordant with the diagnosis. The treatment is directed toward active symptoms of the diagnosis and it demonstrates therapeutic benefits and setbacks.

FIGURE 7.3
Example of Progress Note for John Doe

PROGRESS NOTES

Client: John Doe   Date: 3-6-05

Diagnosis: Major Depression, Dysthymia

Treatment Plan Objectives: (1) Identify sources of depression, (2) Describe/understand conflicts with children

DATA: Current Beck Depression Inventory Score: 29. Previous week 27. Did not complete homework assignment due to "low motivation and too many stressors this week." Client reports a very difficult week in which he missed work 50% of the time. Is complying with Prozac (20 mg. × 2), which he began taking two weeks ago. No noticeable benefits or side effects yet. Very dysphoric over feelings of rejection from family. Often cried when relating feelings of worthlessness. Discussed suicidal contract and steps to follow if feeling suicidal. Gave him another copy of emergency contact phone numbers. Interventions included discussing specific antecedents leading to depressive thoughts and cyclical patterns recurring much of his life. Identified three areas that typically lead to depressed mood; (1) perceived rejection, (2) gives up easily leading to guilt, and (3) thoughts of childhood abuse. Role played having a discussion with his children about his depression and his desire to return to previous functioning. Appeared less depressed during the intervention. Client states that on a scale of 100, usual level of depression is at 85, (baseline was 90, last week was 68, objective is 50). Attended a full session of individual psychotherapy.

ASSESSMENT: A very difficult week in which he seems to be regressing into some negative thought patterns that have usually led to depression. Increased occupational and social impairment. Session seemed helpful in increasing insight and increasing hope.

PLAN: Client will attempt to discuss his depression with his children to increase their understanding that he is not upset with them. Continue keeping journal, which we will review next session. Set up med review with Dr. Anderson.

Time Started: 10:00 A.M.   Time Ended: 10:52 A.M.   Duration: 52 minutes

Type: 90844   Next Session: 3-13-05   Time: 10:00 A.M.

                                                                  Date: 3-6-05

_____
Therapist's Signature and Credentials

Confidentiality Issues and Progress Notes

The HIPAA regulations have clearly changed the nature of accessibility of progress notes. Progress notes in client files are now kept separately from the rest of the file. A separate authorization for records specifically requesting and allowing the progress notes is required. Thus, if an entire file is copied, the progress notes will typically not be included, due to their confidential nature.

This does not mean that progress notes are not subject to audit, nor does it suggest that they are not important. In fact, the progress notes are one of the most crucial documents in a client's file. However, access to them is more limited than the rest of the file due to the personal information that might be disclosed in them.

Some clinicians argue that progress notes should be vague and unrevealing to protect the confidential nature of the session. This argument would be valid if progress notes were meant to disclose confidential material. But well-written progress notes do not need to include potentially damaging confidential information about a client. Some clinicians were trained to produce progress notes that could serve as transcripts of their sessions with clients. These types of progress notes could violate a client's confidentiality if released, and are unnecessary. Other types of progress notes focus on psychological processes rather than the resolution of client problems. These progress notes do provide evidence of personal growth and various processes taking place in the session but do not demonstrate the alleviation of impairments.

Progress notes can be detailed and thorough without sacrificing the client's integrity or confidentiality. A careful look at progress notes requirements reveals that rarely, if ever, do third parties require clinicians to provide a detailed history of client behaviors (outside the session) in progress notes. Historical information is crucial in the course of therapy, but it is not clearly diagnostic or necessary in documentation. Therefore, there is no merit in recording specific aberrant or private behaviors, thoughts, or concerns that could lead to embarrassment or potential legal jeopardy. VandeCreek and Knapp, cited in Soisson et al. (1987) suggest that records should leave out emotional statements, certain personal problems, information about illegal behavior, sexual practices, or other information that may harm the client or others. None of the procedures outlined in this book are designed to raise confidentiality concerns; rather, they are intended to document the efficacy of therapy through evidence of client change.

Other issues arising in progress notes include the client's right to access the information. Although patient records are the property of the provider, the patient controls its dissemination and access to individual records (Soisson et al., 1987). In almost all states, patients have direct access to their records except in cases in which the records could be harmful to the patient.

When patients inspect records and disagree with their content, they have the right to dispute their content and request needed corrections. See Wiger (2005) for clinical forms available designed to fit HIPAA criteria for client's right to disagree or amend client records. See Appendix C for a summary of HIPAA procedures. Such practices increase the clinician's awareness of, and responsibility for, keeping accurate records, which increases accountability in conducting therapy.

Common Problems with Progress Notes

Vagueness

The most common problem with progress notes is vagueness. Progress note statements such as, "discussed emotions," "went over problems," and "practiced communicating," are common but reveal little clinical information and do not document medical necessity of services or treatment progress. Figure 7.4 gives some examples how to make such vague statements clinically relevant.

Progress Notes Unrelated to Treatment Plan Goals

Another red flag for auditors is raised when progress notes do not address the client's diagnosed problem, describe the medical necessity for treatment, or reflect the treatment plan. Figure 7.4 illustrates two examples of progress notes that provide interesting anecdotal information but lack evidence of medical necessity. In addition, the notes raise concerns about potential confidentiality violations and provide little information regarding treatment implications.

The Noncooperative Client

It is difficult to adequately document impairments, progress, and compliance when the client is unwilling to disclose information. This dilemma makes it more difficult to demonstrate the medical necessity for services. For example, a client with paranoia is unlikely to disclose debilitating thoughts and behaviors to a therapist (due to the paranoia). In addition, court-referred clients who deny problems with domestic violence, chemical dependency, perpetrator issues, or other criminal areas for which they are in treatment, tend to admit little or nothing about the behavior in question. Some noncooperative clients claim to have a rapid cure in an effort to terminate therapy.

Although insurance companies will initially reimburse treatment based on a diagnosis, they will only continue paying based on the effectiveness of treatment. Thus, for noncooperative clients for whom it is difficult to properly document the course of treatment, you might do the following:

1. Inform the client that third-party reimbursement depends on accurate diagnosis, client cooperation, therapeutic progress, and documented decreases in impairment. Thus, cooperating in this process is crucial when there is third-party payment. Further inform the client that even if he or she decides to pay cash, the referral source (i.e., a judge or probation officer) may require evidence of progress as part of the rehabilitation process. If the client still refuses to cooperate, other forms of rehabilitation (incarceration, day treatment, and so forth) may be required.

2. Increase the use of collaterals in therapy when the client may be attempting to cooperate but has poor insight. Collaterals may be useful in documenting behavioral changes outside of the counseling sessions. The use of charts and behavioral change graphs provide evidence of progress. For example: "Client's spouse states that he previously consumed at least two quarts of vodka per day. Since the onset of treatment and med. management, he has remained dry. There have been two incidents of temper outbursts (verbal) in the past month. She states that prior to treatment, temper outbursts (physical and verbal) occurred almost daily."

Therapists should be careful about accepting third-party payment for clients who do not want to be in therapy. Poor rates of compliance impede adequate documentation of progress, and it is challenging to elicit information about the client's ongoing impairments. If such cases are audited, there is a possibility that payback will be required. Thus, the clinic could suffer financial losses from seeing such clients if additional efforts are not taken. Worse yet, some third parties contractually prohibit clinics from billing the client for penalties issued due to an audit. Even when back-billing the client is allowed, the chances of collection are low, considering the

FIGURE 7.4
Poorly Documented Progress Note Statements

Example A

Poor example of progress note statement

"Client's deceased uncle, Jay Doe, sexually molested him twenty years ago."

Problems with this statement

1. Does not document how this event affects the client at this time (lacks medical necessity).

2. Implicates the uncle (by name) because it is written as a definitive statement. It is possible that the incident did not take place. In such cases, it is better to quote patient directly. Otherwise, if the client, another relative, or the court were to gain access to the client's file, this potentially unmerited and libelous accusation could be used against the client.

Clinically relevant progress note statement

"Client reports a traumatic incident twenty years ago at age 15, in which he states a deceased relative 'sexually molested' him, currently resulting in recurring nightmares, social withdrawal, and fear of older men."

Why this statement is relevant

The historical incident is alluded to; however, the current symptoms and impairments resulting from the alleged incident are the focus of the progress note. For some, experiencing a severe stressor will not cause a mental health problem; in this case, the effects of stress did cause mental health issues.

Example B

Poorly written progress note statement

"We discussed various problems."

Problems with this statement

1. The statement is vague; thus, there is no way of knowing how this fits the goals and objectives written in the treatment plan.

2. There is no reference to therapeutic techniques or interventions employed in treating the client's problems.

FIGURE 7.4 (Continued)

Clinically relevant progress note statement

"Due to increasing social withdrawal and avoidance at work and other areas, we role-played two ways to socially interact with coworkers. Client appeared tense and said, 'What do I have to offer?' Client appeared more confident after role-playing work situations. He stated that he will attempt these strategies by next session and report level of progress."

Why this statement is relevant

This example provides detail without potentially breaking confidentiality if an outside source had access to the record. It documents that social and occupational impairments are currently taking place and validates dysphoric observations. The effects of treatment strategies were noted, evaluated, and incorporated into the client's life.

Note: When the law requires reporting an incident such as child abuse, intended suicide, intent to harm someone, or taking illegal drugs during pregnancy, it is suggested that the clinician quote what the client stated in the session. The client must be warned of limits to confidentiality prior to receiving services.

therapy may have been conducted a few years prior to the audit. Finally, it is always more difficult to collect payment from clients who did not want to be in therapy in the first place.

SAVING TIME IN WRITING PROGRESS NOTES

Approximately 75% of more than 2,500 therapists surveyed by this author say they write their progress notes after the session. These therapists note that they prefer waiting until after the session ends for the following reasons:

1. "I can't attend to my client if I'm writing notes."
2. "Clients will hold back information or become self-conscious if they believe that I am writing down everything that they say."
3. "They will ask me what I am writing down, become interrupted, and won't concentrate on the session."
4. "I wait until I'm finished with the session so I can integrate the whole picture of what was said."

Others write brief notations during the session and integrate them after the session. Few therapists surveyed claimed to write the bulk of their progress notes during the session. Although there is nothing wrong with any of these procedures, writing progress notes during the session is a time-saver. Imagine a clinician who sees six to eight clients during the day and saves writing progress notes for all clients until the end of the day. The clinician may get a week or two behind and realize there are 30 or more progress notes to write. Now the clinician requires a full day to catch up. Additionally, remembering specifically what took place in each session becomes a mammoth task, typically leading to confabulation.

To avoid having to remember specific details about a session several hours to weeks later and to avoid falling behind, writing progress notes during the session can be a lifesaver. Although the previously mentioned concerns about writing progress notes during the session could occur, with practice, in-session note-taking can be used positively and can enhance empathy. When the clinician nonverbally suggests that what the client says is important (by showing interest when writing things down), clients will often encourage this practice. The time it takes to write a progress note takes only a small fraction of the session time because only the Data section is completed during the session. The Assessment and Plan sections will be completed when the client leaves. For example, in Figure 7.3, the Data section consisted of less than 15 sentences or phrases. Thus, for the session time in Figure 7.3, fewer than one sentence would need to be recorded every 3.5 minutes.

Data are specific pieces of information that do not require continuity or interrelationships; thus it is not necessary for the Data section to read like an ongoing narrative. The data are integrated and used to formulate the Assessment section of the progress note after the session. The Assessment and Plan sections can be written as the client leaves the room. The average time to write these sections is generally less than 5 minutes. If a session lasts 45 minutes and it takes 5 minutes to write the Assessment and Plan sections, it leaves the clinician 10 minutes for a breather before seeing the next client. There is no additional time needed later in the day, and no catch-up time at the clinic is needed. The quality of progress notes is inversely proportionate to the time between the session and writing the progress note.

Another advantage of writing progress notes during the session is that the therapist can more easily quote clients directly and document observations. Much of this information is forgotten, or partially remembered if writing data is deferred for several minutes, hours, or days.

You're well on your way to ensuring that you'll never be held responsible for third-party paybacks. Unfortunately, sometimes even the best planned treatment does not fully alleviate a client's symptoms or impairments in the allotted time frame. In such cases, clinicians must request additional treatment for the client. Convincing third parties that additional therapy is medically necessary is challenging but can be accomplished if the right procedures are followed.

HIGHLIGHTS
of Chapter 7

* ★ Accurate progress notes are crucial because they are the only evidence of progress, therapeutic procedures, and current mental condition.

* ★ Although progress notes are detailed, they do not need to reveal information that might potentially harm the client or others.

* ★ The HIPAA regulations require that a separate request is made for progress notes and that they are kept in a separate file.

* ★ Vague or incomplete progress notes could lead to legal, ethical, or reimbursement issues.

* ★ Well-written progress notes enable a new therapist to quickly resume therapeutic services during times of therapist transition.

* ★ Progress notes reflect the client's progress in specific treatment plan objectives.

* ★ Standard progress note formats, such as SOAP and DAP, follow the scientific method in which the effects of treatment are assessed and a plan is made for future interventions.

* ★ Time can be saved and accuracy can be preserved by writing progress notes during the session.

* ★ Progress notes are not written from a particular theoretical school of thought but, rather, are simply behavioral evidence of the progress from any therapeutic viewpoint.

* ★ Research indicates that therapists can learn new means of writing progress notes when appropriate feedback is available and procedures are simplified.

QUESTIONS

1. Which of the following statements best represents the *Data* from a DAP progress note?

   (a) Client states, "I feel much better this week."

   (b) Therapist states, "Observations suggest improvement in affect."

   (c) Therapist states, "Based on new information, diagnosis is changed to. . . ."

   (d) Therapist states, "Test scores indicate improvements in subjective well-being."

2. Which of the following statements best represents *Assessment* from a DAP progress note?

   (a) Beck Depression Inventory (BDI) score = 21.

   (b) Client cried uncontrollably when role playing saying good-bye to loved one.

   (c) Significant improvements in ability to resolve stressors at home.

   (d) Revise treatment plan objective 3c to. . . .

3. Which of the following statements best represents *Plan* from a DAP progress note?

   (a) The homework assignment for next week is to. . . .

   (b) The homework assignment for this current session was to. . . .

   (c) The homework assignment was detrimental because. . . .

   (d) The homework assignment indicated a significant increase in positive behaviors in the classroom. . . .

4. What is wrong with the following progress note statement that is placed in the Data section? "The client has improved significantly in assertiveness skills."

   (a) It is a good Data statement.

   (b) It adds no significant client information.

   (c) It is too judgmental.

   (d) It is not Data.

5. How might well-written progress notes help protect a therapist from ethical/legal/financial problems?

    (a) They document that appropriate therapeutic and procedural steps were taken prior to a client attempting suicide.

    (b) They demonstrate that the treatment was medically necessary.

    (c) They provide evidence that the treatment provided was concordant with acceptable procedures in the field.

    (d) Each of these.

6. A mental health therapist receives a request for medical information for "The Entire Record." According to HIPAA regulations, what information cannot be sent in this situation?

    (a) Testing

    (b) Progress notes

    (c) Treatment plans

    (d) Diagnostic summary

Answers: 1. a; 2. c; 3. a; 4. d; 5. d; 6. b

8

Documenting the Need for Additional Services

Most insurance and managed care companies require a written request for additional services, once a previously allowed number of services have been utilized. It is not uncommon for a third-party payer to initially authorize two to five sessions and then require documentation that additional services are medically necessary. The content and quality of this written request directly affects the third-party payer's decision to pay for additional services. It is the most crucial piece of documentation material needed to continue services. The therapist's writing and documentation skills are an important part of this aspect of the treatment process. A sample preauthorization request can be found in Appendix A.

Since the third-party case manager does not have direct contact with the client, the only information available is the written mental health records. It is possible for a patient to be in dire need of services, but if the therapist doesn't adequately document this need, services will likely be denied. The third party should not be blamed or held responsible for denying services when documentation does not clearly demonstrate medical necessity. Thus, learning adequate documentation techniques is an obligation to clients, not an unnecessary task or just an additional skill to learn.

Although it might be difficult for some therapists to accept the current documentation requirements, they are a reality, necessary to function within today's standards. On a positive note, those who learn to document well rarely have difficulties obtaining services for clients who need additional services. Effective clinical skills are necessary, but not sufficient, in securing ongoing mental health care for clients; therefore, therapists must be trained and supervised in documentation procedures.

Information commonly requested by a third-party is not difficult to provide if adequate records have been kept. Therapists should not have to rely on their memory about what took place in previous sessions in demonstrating that services are necessary, but, rather, existing documentation that has been kept throughout treatment should be the reference. For example, progress notes and treatment plan updates regularly document medical necessity and the need for continued services. These notations, already documented in the files, may be referred to for documentation when this information is requested by a third party.

There are several types of information typically requested in a preauthorization for additional services request.

- *Mental health diagnosis.* The preauthorization request should include the most current diagnosis. Any diagnosis changes should be incorporated into the treatment plan and clearly explained. In addition, some third-party payers no longer provide payment for certain diagnoses, such as NOS diagnoses, behavioral disorders, Adjustment Disorders, or other diagnoses with a GAF over 60.

- *Service dates and current number of sessions used.* This type of information should correspond with the dates on the progress notes. Third-party payers pay special attention to this information as the number of sessions increases by comparing the number of sessions used to national averages of sessions for various diagnoses. If the number of sessions is significantly more than average, it is important to clearly document any special circumstances that demonstrate a need for additional services. There have been cases in which some managed care companies have not renewed providers' contracts because the clinicians consistently utilized more sessions than the norm.

- *Current mental status and diagnosis documentation.* This information is crucial for obtaining additional services. The key term is *current.* Clinicians must provide an up-to-date validation of the patient's condition. It should reflect progresses and setbacks that have occurred since the onset of treatment. If there is not current documented evidence of a mental health diagnosis, services may be terminated.

- *Current functional impairments.* Since part of the definition of *medical necessity* includes functional impairments, services should be able to continue when the patient continues being impaired but shows progress since the onset of treatment. Thus, the clinician should document and validate the current impairments rather than listing the client's impairments at the onset of treatment.

• *Therapeutic / behavioral progress and regressions.* Some therapists view reporting progress and setbacks as a Catch-22 situation. That is, if clinicians emphasize current impairments and regressions as the evidence that additional services are needed, it will appear that no progress has occurred and make services appear unhelpful on paper. On the other hand, if clinicians emphasize great leaps and progresses, it will appear that no further services are needed.

Both progresses and setbacks should be balanced in the request for additional services report. When progress has occurred but setbacks and impairments still exist, which is often the case, clinicians should provide evidence of both. Ideally, the clinician would document client progress as the result of achieving some treatment plan goals and objectives and document setbacks and continued impairments as areas that have not yet been treated in therapy or as new stressors that have emerged. In this scenario, there is evidence that treatment is working, but more services are necessary to deal with issues not yet treated.

The clinician must exercise ethics in this documentation to prevent painting a different picture of the client on paper than what is actually the case. There may be a temptation to overdocument in order to obtain more services. A good check and balance is to share reports of progress and setbacks with the client.

• *Patient's willingness to accomplish treatment goals and objectives.* Client cooperation is necessary in the counseling process. The preauthorization request should include specific examples of client cooperation in areas such as attending sessions, homework cooperation, therapeutic compliance, and behavioral changes outside the session.

• *Revised or updated treatment plan.* Treatment plans are made to be revised. Without revisions, it is implied that no progress has taken place. Objectives should be periodically revised as clients more closely reach their goals set in the treatment plan.

• *Objective discharge criteria.* Discharge criteria are difficult to determine. Vague statements suggesting discharge criteria such as, "attain 80% of goals," mean very little clinically. The best descriptions are in behavioral terms, suggesting alleviation of functional impairments that led to the medical necessity of services.

HIGHLIGHTS
of Chapter 8

* Most third-party payers request written evidence (preauthorization request) of the effectiveness of treatment in order to reimburse services after a few visits.

* The therapist's documentation and writing skills can directly impact the chances of the client receiving additional services.

* The preauthorization request provides an overview of the client's current mental condition compared to the client's condition at the onset of services, thus measuring clinical effectiveness.

* Both setbacks and progresses of therapy are documented to demonstrate the need for additional services and the benefits of services rendered to date.

* The preauthorization request should demonstrate that treatment has focused on the diagnosis by means of the treatment plan.

QUESTIONS

1. How is it possible for a client who severely needs additional mental health services to be turned down by a case manager from a third-party payer?
   (a) Lack of specific documentation
   (b) Lack of demonstrating medical necessity of services
   (c) Lack of evidence of functional impairments
   (d) All of these

2. When applying for approval for additional client services, why should both progress and setbacks be documented?
   (a) They show both what has been accomplished and what needs to be accomplished in treatment.
   (b) Never document setbacks or lack of progress because it implies that treatment is not effective.
   (c) Never document progresses because it implies that the client is now functioning adequately.
   (d) It doesn't matter which one you document as long as there is evidence that you desire additional services.

3. Why might a client with a diagnosis of Major Depressive Disorder and a GAF of 78 be denied additional services?

  (a) Major Depression is not a serious disorder such as Schizophrenia.

  (b) A client with a GAF of 78 would receive additional services.

  (c) A client with a GAF of 78 is not likely to have significant impairments.

  (d) A client with a diagnosis of Major Depressive Disorder would not have a GAF of 78.

4. Which of the following best represents the best discharge goal?

  (a) Complete eight sessions of psychotherapy.

  (b) Return to work full time.

  (c) Finish discussing disruptive childhood.

  (d) They are all good discharge goals.

5. What is suggested by this statement, "Effective clinical skills are necessary but not sufficient when working with third-party payers."?

  (a) Good therapy skills aren't enough if you don't get along with case managers.

  (b) The third-party payer must know that you work well with people or you will not receive referrals.

  (c) Third-party payers desire that your treatment is effective, not just sufficient.

  (d) Although a therapist might possess excellent clinical skills, their clients may not receive an adequate number of services if the therapist has not learned appropriate documentation skills.

Answers: 1. d; 2. a; 3. c; 4. b; 5. d

A   Appendix

Documented Client Chart for Judy Doe

Appendix A provides additional samples of completed documentation. Some of the formats and procedures are different than those in the text to provide a wider array of examples. For example, the John Doe example throughout the book often emphasizes using specific forms, such as the initial assessment form, in documentation. Documentation can also be narrative as indicated by the examples in this appendix.

DIAGNOSTIC ASSESSMENT REPORT

Name: Judy Doe   DOB: 2-8-82   DOE: 3-5-05

PRESENTING PROBLEM

Signs and Symptoms

Judy Doe, a Caucasian female, age 23, never married, is self-referred for counseling services due to excessive worrying and nervousness. She states that she feels anxious and usually panics whenever she is in public places where she may not be able to get away immediately.

During the interview she appeared to be quite anxious. She often fidgeted, breathed rapidly, and stuttered a few times. She reported having a panic attack in the waiting room prior to the interview.

She began experiencing panic attacks 3 months ago, approximately 1 month after losing her job as a videographer, which she held for 3 years. She currently experiences up to five panic attacks per day, each lasting 20–30 minutes. When she has panic attacks she reports shortness of breath, choking sensations, palpitations, dizziness, chills, and a feeling of doom. Since her first panic attack in public 2 months ago, she refuses to go to public places, such as malls or grocery stores, stating that it is too anxiety-provoking. At home she experiences fewer panic attacks except when the doorbell or phone rings. She will not go out with her friends or relatives and states that she is afraid to apply for another job, noting that she is a "mess-up" and "no one wants to hire a has-been."

History of Present Illness

Judy Doe reports no known family history of mental health treatment. She has never attended a counseling session, nor has she been previously diagnosed with a mental health condition. Most of her life she has been somewhat withdrawn and anxious in public, viewing herself as "shy." She reports that she began feeling increasingly more anxious at work when a "college graduate" was hired in a position similar to hers. The college graduate was eventually promoted in the company due to exceptional work quality. Judy Doe became fairly upset and admits that her work quality suffered from her increased amount of worrying about her job. She began making a greater number of errors and missing work due to headaches and upset stomach. After another "college graduate" was hired, she states her work quality became "poor." She was eventually fired.

Since leaving her job, her anxiety level has increased. She feels incapacitated in her ability to work competitively with people who are more highly trained than her. She worries excessively that if she were able to go back to work that she would just get fired again. One month ago she filled out three job applications and received a phone call for an interview. On the day of the job interview she arrived at the building of the meeting, panicked, and drove home. When she arrived home, she claims to have felt relieved of much of the anxiety.

BIOPSYCHOSOCIAL ASSESSMENT

Judy Doe is the youngest of five children and describes her family as close knit. Her parents have been married for 40 years. She reports that she is from a functional family who treated her "too well" as a child. She describes herself as "daddy's girl" and "the baby of the family." Until she began working full time, her parents took care of all expenses. She lived at home, expense-free, until two years ago.

She currently lives alone in an apartment. Her parents and most of her siblings live within five miles of her. She talks with them on the phone regularly. Two of her sisters visit her at least once per week. About once per month she will visit their homes or her parents in the evening, but may experience panic symptoms in transit. She describes her family as "supportive." Her best friend, whom she has known for over 10 years, recently moved to California due to a job transfer. She has no other close friends.

Educationally, she was in mainstream classes and earned average grades in public school. There were no behavioral or attendance problems in high school. She graduated number 168 out of 350 from high school. She subsequently attended Tech Institute for 1 year of a 2-year program and majored in videography. She left the school after being offered a position at her most recent job where she worked until 3 months ago. Technical school was very difficult for her academically. She stated that she took the videography training only because her friend was going to the program.

As a child she had few friends and was not involved in any school activities or outside events. She was often teased due to her small size and occasional stuttering. Her older siblings often protected her from teasing and ridicule, but she often worried about what would happen if they were not present. She dated a few times as a teenager and as an early adult but was involved in no serious relationships. She states that she is too "reserved" and "afraid" to phone any of her acquaintances or former work associates to enhance her social life, but she wishes she were able to learn how to make friends.

She has not made any new friends since leaving school. She sometimes talks with one of her neighbors on weekends. They have talked about making a trip to Colorado this coming summer, which she describes as "scary." She attends religious services approximately twice per month, which she finds comforting. Her spiritual beliefs and practices are very important to her, and she views them as a definite strength. She describes the people at her place of worship as friendly. She has been asked to join a singles group there but hasn't yet made up her mind because she fears that if no one accepts her, she would feel uncomfortable going to the church.

Prior to developing panic symptoms she enjoyed weekly visits to the zoo by herself. At times she would take her two nieces with her. She played on a neighborhood softball team 2 years ago, but her friend, who urged her to join the team with her, moved away. She did not continue with the team. She still attends family social functions, such as birthday parties, but is not willing to go to events not involving her family. Prior to impairment, she was willing to attend public events if invited by others. She enjoys camping about two times per year with her sisters and their families.

Her last physical evaluation was conducted 6 months ago by Dr. Anderson, of Main Health Clinic. She states that the exam indicated no health concerns. No medications are prescribed. She is allergic to penicillin. Her weight is within normal limits for her height. She was hospitalized once in her life for a tonsillectomy at age 9. She visits the dentist once per year for routine check-ups. She reports no significant physical injuries.

She rarely drinks alcoholic beverages and has never tried illegal drugs. She claims that she has been intoxicated one time in her life, 3 years ago, when she was camping with her sisters. There is no family history of chemical dependence. She has no history of arrests or incarcerations for any reason.

Although she has never been in counseling, she believes it will be helpful because her friend successfully went through counseling following her divorce. She is looking for a female therapist "who understands what it is like being the youngest in a family of high achievers."

MENTAL STATUS EXAM

Clinical Observations

She appeared at the interview neatly dressed and groomed. Her posture and health seemed to be within normal limits. Her nails were very short, as if bitten. She looked her chronological age. There were no unusual mannerisms or gestures. She was alert. Her gait was normal. She sat somewhat rigidly and did not appear relaxed. Initially, she rarely looked at this psychologist, but her eye contact increased as the interview progressed.

Her speech was clear and easily understood but quite soft in volume. She expressed a normal range of vocabulary, pronunciations, and details. At times she was hesitant. Her speech was not mumbled or slurred. There was nothing unusual about her speech.

She was cooperative, answering every question. She seemed somewhat inhibited socially, as evidenced by not initiating interactions, but rather responding only when spoken to. She did not appear to be defensive, guarded, defiant, manipulative, or hostile. She seemed to be interested in the interview process.

Stream of Consciousness

There was no evidence of a thought disorder. She was logical, coherent, and remained on target. No concerns were noticed regarding issues with thought processes, content of thought, thought disturbances, hallucinations, illusions, delusions, or depersonalization. She denied any history of suicidal thoughts, preoccupations, delusions, or detachment.

Affect/Mood

Affective observations included a restricted range of affect. Mobility and intensity of affect were within normal limits. No psychomotor concerns were observed. She appeared to be anxious, as evidenced by often fidgeting with her fingers and hesitancy in her speech. She asked to go to the rest room two times during the interview. She did not appear to be irritable or angry.

She states that she is able to show a normal range of affect toward her family, but not "outsiders." She denies having any anger management issues. When she is upset she usually holds it in rather than expressing it to others. She denies currently feeling depressed but claims to be frustrated with herself due to being unemployed. She does not endorse symptoms suggesting a Depressive Disorder, mania, nor Posttraumatic Stress Disorder.

She currently endorses symptoms and impairments concordant with Panic Disorder with Agoraphobia. Symptoms include abrupt development of heart palpitations, sweating, shortness of breath, chest pain, a feeling of choking, dizziness, and chills. She reports that she has had four panic attacks, each taking place when she had to be in public. She has not been able to feel comfortable in social settings, noting major impairments in which she feels isolated and is not able to apply for a new job.

She further states that for most of her life she only gets involved in activities if she is sure that she will be accepted and liked. In social situations she is often preoccupied with thoughts that people will criticize or reject her. On two occasions she stated that she is "not as good as other people" academically, socially, and on the job. She has taken relatively few risks in her life. She meets criteria for Avoidant Personality Disorder.

Sensorium/Cognition

She was in touch with reality, able to hold a normal conversation, and was oriented × 3. Attention and concentration were within normal limits as evidenced by adequately counting to 40 by threes beginning with 1 and counting backward by sevens from 100 in a normal time period. She repeated six digits forward and four digits backward, which is within the normal range. She correctly spelled the words *stop* and *world* backward.

She recalled three out of three words after 5 minutes and two out of three words after 30 minutes. She remembered the names of previous teachers, historical events in her life, recent meals, and her activities of the past weekend. Short-term, long-term, and immediate memory were intact.

She appeared to have average intelligence. Her level of judgment and abstract thinking were within normal limits. She seems to have appropriate insight into the nature of her concerns, stating that she wants to return to work and learn how to cope with current anxiety.

TESTING

MMPI-2

MMPI-2 results appear to be valid. She finished the testing in a normal time span, responding to every question. Validity scales indicate that she sees herself as experiencing a significant number of problems at this time, which is concordant with the presenting problem.

The basic profiles indicate a 7–0 profile with a slightly elevated 2 scale. People with similar profiles tend to have issues with insecurity, social withdrawal, lack of drive, shyness, and a lack of assertiveness and confidence. The most notable elevation in the profile suggests concerns with anxiety, which is often indicated by longstanding patterns of worrying and poor coping mechanisms. Similar profiles also may indicate concerns with passive aggression.

SUMMARY AND DIAGNOSIS

Judy Doe is self-referred for individual counseling due to panic attacks and resulting social impairment. Symptoms began after losing her job 4 months ago. She further notes symptoms of increased worrying and difficulties going out in public due to panic attacks. She has no counseling history, nor are there any mental health concerns in her family.

She describes her childhood history in positive terms. Being the youngest, her family often took care of most of her needs. Her family is currently supportive. As well, she has one lifelong friend who recently moved out of state. She describes herself as being in average health.

The MSE indicated a normal appearance, speech, and attitude toward this examiner. There was no evidence of a thought disorder. She was fidgety much of the interview and appeared anxious. MMPI-2 testing was concordant with the presenting problems and MSE observations. Memory and concentration were within normal limits. She endorsed symptoms and impairments indicating Panic Disorder with Agoraphobia and Avoidant Personality Disorder.

AXIS I: 300.21   Panic Disorder with Agoraphobia

AXIS II: 302.81   Avoidant Personality Disorder

AXIS III: Defer to Physician

AXIS IV: Unemployment, few friends

AXIS V: GAF = 58 (current)   79 (highest in past year)

_____   3-5-05
Therapist's Signature and Credentials   Date

PROGRESS NOTES

Client: Judy M. Doe   Date: 3-19-05

Diagnosis: Panic Disorder with Agoraphobia, Avoidant Personality Disorder

Objectives for Session: 1) relaxation techniques 2) med. referral 3) anxiety sources

DATA: First therapy session since intake. On time. Signed release of information with Dr. Erikson. Reviewed limits of confidentiality. Reviewed MMPI-2 results, which suggested anxiety, shyness, and concerns with lack of assertiveness. She concurred with results. Client reports a daily average of 5 panic attacks each lasting 20–30 minutes in past week; each time when anticipating going to public places. She states, "I just can't stop them from happening . . . the harder I try, the worse they get . . . I'll never get a job." Insists on keeping therapy sessions in the midafternoon when there is little traffic. Practiced muscle relaxation in three major muscle areas and deep breathing exercises. Initially became more tense when trying to relax. Eventually stated that she felt "more relaxed." Looks forward to daily telephone calls from her family, stating that she "needs them." Discussed feelings of dependency and need for approval. She replied, "That's what families are for." Attended a full session of individual psychotherapy. Topics included test results, relaxation, and family dynamics.

ASSESSMENT: Slight increase in number of panic attacks. Somewhat pessimistic about employment at this time. Seemed tense in learning relaxation techniques; eventually soothed. Supportive family but concerns with dependency. Her attempts to curtail panic attacks increase anxiety.

PLAN: Will practice two relaxation techniques daily. Will write diary of feelings after talking with family on telephone. Next session: Continue relaxation training and family dynamics, review diary.

Time Started: 1:30 P.M.   Time Ended: 2:15 P.M.   Duration: 45 minutes

Type: 90840   Next Session: 3-26-05   Time: 1:30 P.M.

                                                        3-19-05
_____   _____
Therapist's Signature and Credentials   Date

PROGRESS NOTES

Client: Judy M. Doe   Date: 3-26-05

Diagnosis: Panic Disorder with Agoraphobia, Avoidant Personality Disorder

Objectives for Session: 1) relaxation techniques 2) family dynamics

DATA: Session 2. Med. evaluation will be this week with Dr. Erikson. Compliant with homework assignment. Has not looked into any job possibilities. Reports four panic attacks this week in which she tried repeating relaxation techniques. Although these techniques did not stop them, they may have decreased duration of attacks from 20–30 minutes to about 15 minutes on average. Stated that she feels helpless during an attack and "always" phones home when in distress. Journaling notations indicate relief of stress when in contact with family. Brought up increasing resentments toward family due to "taking care of me . . . I want to make my own mistakes." Family will be incorporated as future collaterals in treatment. Reviewed and refined two relaxation techniques. Used guided imagery techniques in imagining going to grocery store. Some resistance but followed through. Gave her a handout of assertiveness training group at Main Hospital. Attended full session.

ASSESSMENT: Cooperative and motivated to change but has difficulties acknowledging dependence on family for stress alleviation. Guided imagery techniques were helpful. Deep breathing seems more effective than muscle relaxation at this time. Somewhat reluctant to join group therapy at this time.

PLAN: Assigned reading of "Take Control of Your Anxiety." Client will discuss collateral sessions with family parents and two sisters. No changes in objectives.

Time Started: 1:30 P.M.   Time Ended: 2:15 P.M.   Duration: 45 minutes

Type: 90840   Next Session: 4-2-05   Time: 1:30 P.M.

                                                      3-26-05
_____
Therapist's Signature and Credentials   Date

REQUEST FOR ADDITIONAL SERVICES

Client: Judy M. Doe   Date: 4-12-05

Primary Diagnosis: 300.21   Panic Disorder with Agoraphobia

Other Diagnosis: 302.81   Avoidant Personality Disorder

Hours Requested: 10: 6 individual, 4 conjoint

History: No prior mental health treatment, self or family. Describes self as typically shy and nervous prior to onset of panic symptoms. No close friends. Lost job held for 3 years 4 months ago. Since losing job experiences panic attacks when leaving the house. Too anxious/fearful to apply for jobs.

Diagnostic Features: Panic symptoms include shortness of breath, choking feeling, palpitations, feelings of doom, dizziness, and chills. Onset: 1-05. Frequency: 3/day. Duration: 20–30 minutes. Severity: moderate. History of social avoidance, with increasing severity.

Current Stressors/Impairments: Currently unemployed and under financial stress. Increasing level of panic attacks, anxiety, and worrying causing inability to go on job interviews. No social supports outside of her family, on whom she is dependent. Avoiding most people.

Progresses/Setbacks in Therapy: Client reports decreased duration of panic attacks due to relaxation techniques. Gaining insight into family dynamics leading to dependency. Considering assertiveness group. Cooperative, motivated to change. Somewhat reluctant to try new techniques.

Treatment Plan Revisions: No revisions at this point. Presently working on current objectives.

Referrals/Medications: Referred to Dr. Erikson for physical exam and med. evaluation. Appointment on 4-22. No Hx of meds. Signed release of information with Dr. Erikson.

Discharge Plans: 80% of treatment plan goals met. Reduce number and duration of panic attacks to <2 per week lasting less than 10 minutes. Learn relaxation and coping techniques to control anxiety. Regularly search for employment and attend job interviews. Decrease dependency on family. Increase social interactions and assertiveness, such as initiating at least one social interaction daily.

_____	4-12-05 _____
Therapist's Signature and Credentials	Date

PROGRESS NOTES

Client: Judy M. Doe   Date: 7-19-05

Diagnosis: Panic Disorder with Agoraphobia, Avoidant Personality Disorder

Objectives for Session: 1) Review of all treatment plan objectives 2) Increase social contacts

DATA: Session 9. Reviewed treatment plan objectives to date. 1) has become proficient in muscle relaxation, 2) has reduced number and duration of panic attacks—currently averaging two panic attacks weekly, duration 10–12 minutes, 3) receiving medications from MD, 4) difficulties following through with implementing new coping mechanisms, 5) has initiated approximately one social contact daily, but with people she knew previously. No initial contacts with unknown people. Discussed revisions of objectives. Appeared less anxious than previous sessions. Has attended assertiveness group 3 weeks in a row; beginning to feel safe. Experiencing some stress when attempting to assert own opinions toward family. Continued exploring family dynamics and social avoidance issues. Has applied for two jobs in past week; did not panic but experienced anxiety. One interview later this week.

ASSESSMENT: Most treatment plan objectives on target for date. Soon ready to work again. Medications effective; no side effects. Continued difficulties with assertiveness, social avoidance, and social withdrawal.

PLAN: See revised treatment plan. Will schedule approximately six more sessions. Homework to introduce self to at least five people this week.

Time Started: 1:30 P.M.   Time Ended: 2:15 P.M.   Duration: 45 minutes

Type: 90840   Next Session: 7-26-05   Time: 1:30 P.M.

_____   7-19-05_____

Therapist's Signature and Credentials   Date

B Appendix

Overview of Outcome Measures

The material in Appendix B provides an overview of outcomes, but it is not intended to present comprehensive outcomes training. See Wiger and Solberg (2001) for training in several aspects of outcomes.

Prior to the late 1970s to early 1980s, mental health services represented only 3% to 4% of the health care dollars spent by employers. But mental health costs have skyrocketed by as much as 30% to 40% per year, and mental health services grew from 4% to nearly 35% of the money spent on health care by the early 1990s (Lyons, Howard, O'Mahoney, & Lish, 1997). To reduce costs, services were limited and subject to increasing guidelines for approval. Outcome measures have increasingly developed to help determine the most efficient means of providing quality services. The basic questions being asked in outcomes measures are, "What evidence is there that psychotherapy is working?" and, "What types of mental health services work most effectively for whom?" As outcomes measures research has developed, issues have arisen regarding what needs to be measured and how it will be helpful. Table B.1 provides eight principles of outcomes measurement.

Browning and Browning (1996), developers of the Browning Outcomes Survey Scale (BOSS) state that the best judge of therapeutic outcomes is the person who received services; therefore, much of outcomes measurement is based on self-report. The BOSS comes in three versions: intake, discharge, and 6-month follow-up. Both Likert ratings for quantification and comment sections for quality are included for each of several dimensions. The authors suggest sharing the findings regularly with case managers in either a summary format or by providing a copy of the instrument. Copies of the BOSS are available from Duncliff's International at 1-800-410-7766.

Lyons et al. (1997) suggest three dimensions of satisfaction based on the Rand Corporation for the Medical Outcomes Study (Ware & Hays, 1988). These dimensions include technical quality, competence, interpersonal quality, access, and availability and choice of services. Examples of areas to assess are found in Figure B.1.

TABLE B.1

Principles of Outcome Measurement

What to Measure

Principle 1.   Define the goals and objectives of the service and measure their clinical aspects. Do not measure what is irrelevant to these goals and objectives.

Principle 2.   Determine what is important to consumers, providers, and customers of the services, and attempt to include these in the measurement.

Principle 3.   Determine what is possible and practical to measure. Try not to overreach in any single effort. Multiple short-term studies are often more feasible and of greater value than comprehensive but overly complicated long-term efforts.

How to Measure

Principle 4.   Know the existing measurement choices. Do not create a new measure needlessly. Choose measures with relevant databases that provide norms and benchmarks against which to assess consumers.

Principle 5.   Decide who should provide assessments of clinical status based on the nature of the treatment and the characteristics of the consumers served.

Principle 6.   Choose measures that are reliable, valid, brief, and easy to use.

When to Measure

Principle 7.   Always measure at the earliest possible time. Assessment at the initiation of treatment is essential for estimating change.

Principle 8.   Measure again on a fixed schedule, particularly when the end of treatment is not predictable. This method allows statistical options for estimating end-of-treatment clinical status.

Source: The Measurement & Management of Clinical Outcomes in Mental Health (p. 36) by Lyons et al., 1997. New York: John Wiley & Sons. Reprinted by permission.

The material in Figure B.1 is not intended to be a formal outcomes questionnaire; rather, it provides helpful guidelines regarding the type of information that can aid in an outcomes assessment. The formatting of the questions can range from Yes-No questions, to a Likert scale, to a narrative.

TYPES OF DATA USED IN DOCUMENTING OUTCOMES

Yes-No Questions

Yes-No questions in outcomes measurement are calculated by the percentage of survey items either endorsed as "Yes" or "No" (or similar contrasting terms such as Agree/Disagree, Positive/Negative, or Improved/Declined, etc.). For example, items such as, "Did your therapist seem to listen to your

FIGURE B.1
Suggested Dimensions of Client Satisfaction in Outcomes Studies

Examples of Technical Quality Dimensions

Were the educational materials helpful?

Were the medications explained to you?

Did you understand the possible side effects of your prescription when you finished your visit?

Was the equipment in good working condition?

Were the program's policies explained to you?

Was the billing procedure accurate?

Examples of Competence Dimensions

Did you feel your therapist was qualified to provide the care you needed?

Did you find the hospital staff sufficiently well trained?

Did your therapist discuss your treatment plan with you in a manner that you could understand?

Was the intake worker able to provide sufficient information about the available services?

To what degree were you confident that the program staff were skilled in their professions?

Examples of Interpersonal Competence Dimensions

Did you feel that your case manager was concerned with your well-being?

Did you experience your therapist as warm and supportive?

Did you feel comfortable talking to program staff?

Did program staff listen to you when you had a question or concern?

Did you feel that your problems were being taken seriously?

Examples of Access to Care Dimensions

Was the geographical location of your therapist convenient?

How long did you have to wait to see the crisis worker? How did you feel about the wait?

How many days passed between the time you called to request services and when you were able to see your therapist? How did you feel about this amount of time?

How did you feel about the costs of your treatment?

How did you feel about the copayment?

How did you experience the process of obtaining treatment?

Did you have any concerns about the confidentiality of the service? Were these concerns communicated and addressed?

Source: The Measurement & Management of Clinical Outcomes in Mental Health (pp. 50–53) by Lyons et al., 1997. New York: John Wiley & Sons. Reprinted by permission.

concerns?" requests either a positive or negative response, with no in-between choices. These include specific answers from a particular client and an analysis of how several clients answered various questions. Outcomes measures from 100 clients might indicate that 72% of clients surveyed agree that their therapists listened to their concerns, and 28% did not agree.

The main problem with Yes-No questions is that they assume a person totally agrees or totally disagrees with the statement. A "No" answer implies that the therapist did not listen at all to the client's concerns, whereas a "Yes" answer implies no problems in this area. When a client fills out a questionnaire with this format (called *ipsative*), there is no place for partial agreement. That is, if the client believes that the therapist listened some of the time, there is a dilemma as to how to answer the question. Results allow the researcher to have a general idea of outcome measures, but the degree is unknown.

Likert Scale Ratings

Likert ratings provide answers on a continuum in which a degree of agreement or disagreement with a statement is possible. For example, in the previous outcomes measures question, "Did your therapist seem to listen to your concerns?" the wording would have to be changed to a statement, rather than a question, because a level of agreement is needed. For example, a Likert rating scale could be incorporated for the statement, "The therapist seemed to listen to my concerns." Likert ratings are numerical ratings in which the client's level of agreement is analyzed. When the highest point on the scale is an odd number, there is a midpoint in which the client is neutral in the response. A Likert scale of 1–7 is commonly used. Some Likert scales use an even number of items, in which there is no mid or neutral point. Data from Likert ratings, such as those found in Figure B.2, can be used for several possible outcome measures.

Figure B.3 provides an example of Likert rating items.

FIGURE B.2
Use of Likert Ratings in Outcomes Measurement

1. Pretreatment, midtreatment, discharge, and posttreatment scores
2. Treatment variables (type of, number of sessions)
3. Clinician variables (style, empathy, background, education, experience)
4. Diagnosis (chronic, acute, onset, duration, intensity of symptoms, impairments)
5. Demographic variables (age, race, socioeconomic status, previous treatment)
6. Treatment/medication compliance (attendance, compliance in homework, meds, interventions)

FIGURE B.3
Example of Likert Scale Items in Outcome Measures

Please circle the response which most closely indicates your level of agreement or disagreement with the following statements.

Highly Disagree 1	Moderately Disagree 2	Slightly Disagree 3	Neutral 4	Slightly Agree 5	Moderately Agree 6	Highly Agree 7

"I was given choices about my treatment."

| 1 | 2 | 3 | 4 | 5 | 6 | 7 |

"The therapist explained the benefits and risks of therapy to me."

| 1 | 2 | 3 | 4 | 5 | 6 | 7 |

"I was treated with respect and dignity by the therapist."

| 1 | 2 | 3 | 4 | 5 | 6 | 7 |

"The therapist listened to my concerns."

| 1 | 2 | 3 | 4 | 5 | 6 | 7 |

"The treatment plan was clearly explained to me."

| 1 | 2 | 3 | 4 | 5 | 6 | 7 |

"Services were performed in a time-efficient manner."

| 1 | 2 | 3 | 4 | 5 | 6 | 7 |

"The clinic's policies were clearly explained to me."

| 1 | 2 | 3 | 4 | 5 | 6 | 7 |

"The counseling was directed toward helping my problem areas."

| 1 | 2 | 3 | 4 | 5 | 6 | 7 |

"I was satisfied with the counseling I received."

| 1 | 2 | 3 | 4 | 5 | 6 | 7 |

"The services I received were helpful."

| 1 | 2 | 3 | 4 | 5 | 6 | 7 |

"I would return to the therapist for services in the future if needed."

| 1 | 2 | 3 | 4 | 5 | 6 | 7 |

USE OF OUTCOME DATA

Ultimately, outcome measures most benefit the client by providing evidence of the most cost-effective treatment by the most qualified professionals. The process of collecting and utilizing outcomes data helps make this possible.

On an individual level, outcomes data can be useful to the client/consumer as a motivator that therapy is working and that it is cost-effective.

Properly conducted outcome studies within may result in the therapist changing interventions that are not helpful and maintaining interventions that result in progress. Third-party payers benefit in that they are assured that their funds are being used to benefit clients who have paid for such services. When outcome measures indicate lack of progress it provides a flag that current interventions are not alleviating the client's impairments. In general, third-party payers request individual outcome measures on a client-by-client basis. Outcomes training found in Wiger and Solberg (2001) teaches how to collect outcomes data in all aspects of treatment such as the interview, treatment plan, progress notes, and through standardized outcome measures.

Accrediting agencies such as JCAHO and CARF mandate outcome measures. Outcomes measurement in mental health is in its infancy. Most books on this topic have been published in the past 10 years. A few examples include Lyons et al. (1997), Ogles, Lambert, and Masters (1996), Sperry, Brill, Howard, and Grisson (1996), Howard, Orlinsky, and Lueger (1994), and Orlinsky and Howard (1986).

C Appendix

Overview of HIPAA Guidelines in Mental Health Settings
(from Wiger, 2005)

The following information is not intended to constitute comprehensive HIPAA training, but, rather, it briefly summarizes the rationale for the guidelines. The HIPAA guidelines specifically state that there are no approved training courses, and consumers are cautioned to be aware of programs that present themselves as such.

The U.S. Department of Health and Human Services (HHS) implemented the Health Insurance Portability and Accountability Act (HIPAA) in 1996. HIPAA is designed to both protect people's health information and provide standardized means of regulating the flow of information. Its major purposes are to (a) protect individuals from losing their health insurance when they change jobs, (b) allow medical savings accounts, (c) help prevent abuse and fraud, and (d) simplify health insurance administrative procedures. Prior to HIPAA regulations there were about 400 different formats of electronic claims submission in the United States. Providers must adhere to standard codes, and are not allowed to modify or use additional code sets; thus uniformity and cost savings are assured. Complete rules may be found on the Office of Civil Rights (OCR) website at http://www.hhs.gov/ocr/hipaa.

HIPAA's "Privacy Rule" refers to the standards of disclosure of "protected health information" by "covered entities" (those subject to the regulations). The covered entities include health care clearinghouses, health plans, and health care providers who transmit health information electronically or use billing services that transmit electronically.

The covered entity must have a written contract with each business associate to safeguard the protected health information. All individually identifiable health information held or transmitted by a covered entity or its business associate (nonmember of covered entity's workforce, who has access to protected health information, e.g., billing service, utilization review) requires this contract. The OCR website provides a sample at http://www.hhs.gov/ocr/hipaa/contractprov.html.

Healthcare providers who are covered entities must disclose protected health information in two broad situations. These include providing the information to (a) the individual (or personal representative) who requests their records, and (b) to HHS in a compliance action. The covered entity may disclose protected health information without the individual's consent in the following situations. It may be disclosed as follows:

1. The individual who is the subject of the protected health information (i.e., client, patient) is not required to authorize information sent to self.

2. Protected health care information that is used in the normal operation of providing services, consultation, and referral does not need a specific authorization (treatment, payment, and health care operations).

3. Payment operations, such as premiums, determination of benefits, and billing services, are not subject to an authorization.

4. Health care operations such as quality improvement, case management, competency assurance activities (e.g., credentialing, accreditation), audits, reviews, insurance functions, business development, and administrative activities may use a "limited data set" in which records are "deidentified" (patient information does not include identifying information, such as name, social security number, or other specific identifiers).

5. The public interest can override confidentiality in situations such as when the health, welfare, or safety of others may be in jeopardy. Certain civil operations such as court orders, crimes, and essential government services necessary for the public's best interest, do not require an individual's authorization for disclosing protected health information.

The covered entity is required to treat the individual's "personal representative" with the same rights as the individual in matters of disclosure. The personal representative is legally allowed to make health care decisions for the individual, except in cases of suspected abuse. In general, parents are the personal representatives of their minor children and have access to protected health information, except in cases where the law would allow discretion on behalf of the licensed health care professional.

DISCLOSURE OF INFORMATION

A written authorization from the individual (or authorized representative) to the covered entity must precede a release of protector health care information. The content of the authorization must be in specific terms, written in plain language. The authorization must designate which information is being requested (rather than asking for an entire file), include an expiration date, and describe the individual's right to revoke the authorization.

In most cases, an individual must consent to disclose psychotherapy progress notes. Exceptions include ongoing psychotherapy with the originator of the progress notes, training, legal matters brought on by the individual, legal reasons, and for the public interest.

The practice of routinely requesting an individual's entire record is discouraged. The Privacy Rule requires the limiting of the amount of information disclosed to the "minimum necessary." The covered entity is required to develop and implement policies to set guidelines for determining what is the minimum amount of information necessary for the intended purpose of the disclosure. Policies and procedures regarding which persons or categories of persons in the covered entity's workforce will have access to which level of protected health information in order to adequately perform their duties. When covered entities receive requests for specific information, it can be assumed that the level of information requested is reasonable.

Covered entities are required to provide a notice of privacy practices that describes people's rights to privacy, the duties of the covered entity, and the complaint process. This notice must be distributed to the individual at their first encounter (e.g., office, electronic, mailing). It must be posted in a prominent space where the individual can read it. The covered entity must make reasonable efforts to obtain the individual's signature that the notice was received.

The covered entity has the right to review their medical records (designated health set). However, the covered entity may choose to not disclose (a) psychotherapy progress notes, (b) information from legal proceedings, and (c) laboratory results, when it is deemed as not being in the individual's best interest.

Individuals have a right to amend information in their protected health information when they consider the information to be inaccurate or incomplete. If the information is amended, reasonable efforts must be made to provide the revised information to those identified by the individual as in need of the information and to others who rely on this information for treatment. When the request for an amendment is denied, the individual has the right to make a statement of the disagreement that will be included in the record.

Glossary

Abstractive capacity A person's ability to think abstractly. Children often think concretely, whereas an average adult is able to think conceptually rather than perceptually.

> *Documentation examples:*
>
> In the MSE, the clinician often asks the client to interpret various proverbs that could be interpreted either concretely or abstractly. An abstract interpretation of "The early bird catches the worm," could be, "Those who get up early have the best opportunities," whereas a concrete interpretation is generally more literal. A child or an adult with limited intelligence or brain damage might interpret this proverb as, "Birds catch worms in the morning." Tests of abstract thinking may also indicate signs of a thought disorder. Responses such as, "Birds who fly never die if they eat a worm every day to keep the doctor away," generally indicate concerns beyond the normal range of concrete vs. abstract thought patterns.

Accreditation An external review process in which a provider of services has been approved by an outside source that sets acceptable standards of performance in which others can make decisions about the provider.

Activity level A series of observations in the MSE including notations such as a client's mannerisms, gestures, degree of relaxation versus tenseness, eye contact, vigilance, gait, degree of boredom, attentiveness, and body movements.

> *Documentation examples:*
>
> Increased activity level: "Increased activity level was observed as evidenced by several body movements, tenseness, often getting out of the chair, and hypervigilance."

Decreased activity level: "The client's activity level appeared decreased as evidenced by low attention span, masked facies, psychomotor retardation, and slow speech."

Affective observations   The client's degree of affect (emotions) as observed by the clinician. See appropriateness of affect, intensity of affect, mobility of affect, range of affect, and predominant mood.

Documentation examples:

Depressed mood: "The client appeared dysphoric as evidenced by blunted affect, low mobility of affect, restricted range of affect, few facial expressions, and crying at times."

Anxious mood: "The client appeared anxious. Observations included low eye contact, sweating, irritability, and excessive worrying."

Appearance   Objective observations made by the clinician describing the client's grooming, manner of dress, hygiene, posture, health, demeanor, and apparent age.

Documentation examples:

Appearance suggesting depressed mood: "Client appeared at the interview appearing dysphoric as evidenced by disheveled hair, slumped posture, beard stubble, and lack of facial expression."

Appearance suggesting mania: "The client wore extremely bright clothing not suggestive of his usual appearance. Activity level was increased."

Appearance suggesting thought disorder, Dementia, or possible substance abuse: "The client appeared at the interview with a soiled winter coat (in the summertime), mismatched socks, and no shoe laces. There was a strong body odor. He appeared to be in poor health, looking approximately 15 years older than his chronological age."

Appropriateness of affect   Affective observations indicating the concordance between the client's stated mood, speech, and ideas.

Documentation examples:

Example 1: "Although the client stated that she was severely depressed and suicidal, she often spoke in an animated manner, joked, and seemed to be somewhat flirtatious."

Example 2: "The client sat in the interview calmly, appearing relaxed, but stated that he was extremely worried and having panic symptoms."

Assessment   The continuous process in integrating clinical data to form an objective clinical opinion. Assessment data in mental health comes from sources such as observations, information gathered from others, and standardized testing. Simply reporting data is not an assessment. Generally, the more effectively the data is integrated, the better the assessment. Assessment information is used to determine the most appropriate treatment for the client.

Associated symptoms Symptoms that are often linked to a mental health disorder but not used in validating a diagnosis because they are also prevalent in several disorders.

> Examples of associated symptoms: Social withdrawal, difficulties coping, low self-esteem, fatigue, irritability, difficulty concentrating.

Attention or **attention span** The ability to cognitively focus on a stimulus when in an aroused state. Common MSE tasks to assess attention include incrementally repeating numbers (digit span) forward and backward. Other indices include the examiner's observations of the client's level of attention in holding a conversation.

> *Documentation examples:*
>
> Low attention span: "Client's attention span appeared to be significantly below average, as evidenced by asking to have several questions repeated, repeating 3 digits forward and 2 digits backward, and often staring into space."

Attitude toward examiner The client's general attitude observed during the interview. Descriptions include aspects such as cooperation, level of interest, guardedness, defiance, humor, defensiveness, evasiveness, suspiciousness, manipulative, and level of historical information provided. The validity of the interview is affected by this variable.

> *Documentation examples:*
>
> Negative attitudinal concerns: "Attitudinal concerns were noted during the interview in which the client made several defiant comments, refused to supply background information, made several derogatory comments, and stated that he does not trust anyone with a tie."
>
> Positive attitude: "The client was cooperative, answered every question, provided detailed historical information, and seemed interested throughout the interview."

Axis I: Mental Disorders A *DSM* diagnosis describing a mental health diagnosis. All mental health diagnoses in the *DSM-IV-TR* are considered Axis I, except Personality Disorders and Mental Retardation.

Axis II: Personality Disorders and Mental Retardation *DSM* diagnoses of Personal Disorders and Mental Retardation.

Axis III: Physical Conditions and Disorders *DSM* diagnoses of a physical nature. These may or may not have a bearing on mental disorders. Mental health professionals generally defer this diagnosis to a physician or refer to information received from a physician.

Axis IV: Psychosocial and Environmental Problems A *DSM* Axis that includes a listing of current stressors in the client's life that may be contributing to mental health issues.

Axis V: Global Assessment of Functioning An overall *DSM* assessment of the client's current level of functioning on a 100 point scale. It also allows for noting changes in functioning over a period of time.

Biopsychosocial assessment An ongoing assessment of the client's biological, psychological, and social functioning.

CARF Commission of Accreditation of Rehabilitation Facilities is a private accrediting agency for health care organizations designed to improve the quality of care from member organizations to the public.

Clang associations A type of loose association in which statements are interrelated by their sounds, rather than meaning.

> *Example:* "I went to Brent at Trent and spent the rent in a dent by a tent."

Clinical observations Any observations made by the therapist regarding client behaviors. Typical observations include aspects such as affect, appearance, activity level, speech, and attitude toward examiner.

Cognition Mental processing of information involving memory and thinking. Mental status observations include indices such as the client's apparent contact with reality, orientation × 3, attention, and concentration.

Collateral information Background and clinical information about the client provided by other people such as other professionals, family members, and significant others.

Compulsions Repeated physical or mental acts viewed as not useful to the client. Examples include behaviors such as repeatedly washing hands, locking doors, checking that appliances are turned off, or other excessive behaviors of clinical significance.

Concentration The ability to focus attention over a period of time. The MSE measures of concentration typically include tasks such as counting by serial threes beginning with 1, or counting backward by sevens from 100.

Documentation examples:

Poor concentration: "Client's concentration seemed to be significantly below average, as evidenced by not being able to count by serial threes beginning with 1 and sometimes forgetting the topic of a question asked after providing only part of the answer."

Adequate concentration: "The client's level of concentration appeared to be within normal limits as evidenced by rapidly counting backward from 100 by sevens in a normal time period, making zero errors.

Confidentiality   An agreement between the therapist and client that the information disclosed to the therapist will not be shared with other people without the client's consent. State laws impose certain limits of confidentiality that should be disclosed to the client prior to receiving services.

DAP notes   A progress note format in which three distinct sections are outlined including Data, Assessment, and Plan.

Data   Specific information, such as observations, test scores, client statements, and collateral information, that is used to form an assessment.

Delusions   Untrue or incorrect beliefs that are not religiously or culturally approved. Contrary evidence does not change these beliefs. Common types of delusions include paranoid, grandeur, nihilistic, and somatic.

Depersonalization   A subjective experience of feeling detached or outside of one's body or in a dream.

Derailment   A loosening of associations depicted by unrelated thoughts. Clients jump from one thought to another without a logical transition, which is likened to a train jumping off the rail.

> *Example:* A client might say, "I balloon never before Sally pepper chair over there."

Discharge   The time in which the clinician or treatment center no longer holds responsibility for the care of the patient. Generally a discharge summary report accompanies discharge.

Echolalia   Recurring repetitions of another person's speech.

Effectiveness   The level in which clinical interventions and care are provided in accordance to the current level of knowledge and practice in the field. Greater effectiveness produces greater outcomes and a lower level of risk.

Efficacy   The level of positive outcomes for the client resulting from treatment.

Efficiency   The correspondence between the resources used in providing treatment and the outcomes of treatment. Sometimes called cost-effectiveness ratio or cost/benefits ratio in which the results of treatment are compared to the cost of treatment.

Essential symptoms   *DSM-IV-TR* symptoms that must be prevalent for a diagnosis to be made. Also called core symptoms.

Euphoria   An elevated normal mood state. Not a manic state. Often described as a state of happiness.

Euthymic   A normal range of mood states.

Flight of ideas   A rapid succession of interconnected ideas in which the client's conversation changes quickly. The topic of conversation may change from sentence to sentence, but logic is retained.

Goals   The client's overall desired outcomes from therapy. The endpoints of various objectives in therapy.

Hallucinations   Perceptual disturbances without corresponding outside stimulation. Hallucinations are associated with all five of the senses. They are often associated with psychosis.

HIPAA   The Health Insurance Portability and Accountability Act, created in 1996 by the U.S. Department of Health and Human Services, is designed to both protect people's health information and provide standardized means of regulating the flow of information.

Health Maintenance Organization (HMO)   A source that arranges or provides coverage of health services to members.

Illusions   A misperception or distortion of an outside stimulus.

> *Example:* Trees blowing in the wind may be perceived as demons or giants.

Immediate memory   Memories recently stored.

> *Example:* In the MSE the clinician may ask the client to remember three unrelated words after 5- and 30-minute intervals.

Impairments   Areas in a person's life that are not functional; therefore, treatment is *medically necessary*. Also called functional impairments. Commonly documented areas of impairment include social, occupational, affective, physical, and academic.

> *Example:* "Due to increased irritability and aggression over the past year, the client currently has no friends or social supports. He has not

been involved in any social activities for several months and is becoming increasingly more withdrawn, resulting in social impairment."

Intensity of affect   The strength of affective expression that is often put on a continuum from mild to strong.

JCAHO   The Joint Commission on Accreditation of Healthcare Organizations is private accrediting agency for health care organizations designed to improve the quality of care from member organizations to the public.

Loose associations   The absence or loss of logical connectedness in speech. Speech transitions seem to have little association.

> *Example:* "I like bananas because they taste good and children walk to school."

Malingering   The intentional presentation of signs and symptoms of a mental disorder. It is generally intended to achieve some sort of gain or to avoid unpleasant circumstances.

Medicaid   A federally funded, state administered program that provides healthcare benefits to people with low income.

Medical model   The medical model views mental health service delivery as treating pathology in which documentation consists of symptoms reduction.

Medical necessity   Mental health services are considered medically necessary when significant dysfunction or impairments exist that result from a diagnosable mental disorder. Services are needed to either restore functioning or prevent deterioration.

Medical record   The client's record of documented clinical information related to services provided.

Mobility of affect   The rate in which a person moves from one type of affect to another. For example, if a client moves rapidly from dysphoria to euphoria, it would be described as lability or increased mobility. Little or no mobility is described as constricted or fixed.

Mood   The client's description of his or her current or usual affective state.

Mood Disorder   Mood Disorders are classified as diagnoses in mania, depression, or both. Also called affective disorder.

Neologisms   New or nonsense words used by the client but not recognized as unusual words.

> *Example:* "The cirplexanity of the situation leads to additional recountations."

Objectives   Objectives are sequential steps by which treatment plan goals are met. Each objective, when attained, is revised to more closely reach the goal.

Obsessions   Intrusive and persistent unwanted thoughts that will not go away despite attempts to suppress them and despite knowledge that the thought is not reality based or is out of proportion to reality.

Orientation   A person's ability to understand his or her connection in relation to aspects such as time, place, and person. In the MSE, the clinician generally states that the person is "oriented times 3" when referring to orientation in all three areas.

Outcomes   The empirical results of a course of treatment in which outcomes criteria set by the reviewer are evaluated.

Poverty of speech   The client's speech has little depth or meaningful information. Sometimes little is spoken, whereas others may speak full sentences.

Preoccupation   A recurrent theme, thought, or idea often prevalent in the client's conversations or thoughts.

> *Example:* "They're evil. This world is wicked. I dream about the awful things happening. My friends, family, and everyone . . . they're all evil. I always know when the bad people are coming."

Presenting problem   The client's statement of the problem area or reason for seeking services. It is not a diagnosis, but problem areas will be assessed to help determine the need for services.

Prognosis   The clinician's opinion as to the probability of the client leaving services with a positive outcome. Typical descriptions include poor, marginal, guarded, moderate, good, and excellent. It is common for the clinician to also include qualifiers, such as compliance, to the prognosis for areas such as medications, treatment, or changes in areas such as behaviors or education.

Provisional diagnosis   A diagnosis qualifier that is given when there is yet insufficient information to warrant a full diagnosis.

Psychomotor agitation   A behavioral observation in the MSE in which the client appears to have difficulties sitting still, attending to tasks, or appears tense.

Psychomotor retardation   A behavioral observation in the MSE in which the client's movements and other behaviors are slow.

Range of affect   The client's ability to express a variety of affective responses in various situations. Descriptors are often depicted as normal, restricted, blunted, or flat.

Recent memory   Memories of recent events in the client's life. MSE questions, such as the client's memory of recent meals and events of the past weekend, are typically asked.

Remote memory   Memories of historical events in the client's life. MSE questions, such as the name of the street they grew up on, previous teachers' names, or asking someone born prior to the mid-1950s what they were doing when they heard that President Kennedy was shot.

Signs   Characteristics of a mental disorder are those that are observed objectively by the clinician.

SNAPs   An acronym for the client's strengths, needs, abilities, and preferences, in which these characteristics are incorporated into the client's treatment.

SOAP notes   A progress note format in which four distinct sections are outlined including Subjective, Objective, Assessment, and Plan.

Somatoform Disorder   A variety of physical disorders with emotional origins.

Symptoms   Characteristics of a mental disorder reported by the affected individual.

Third-party payer   A source such as an individual, organization, or government entity that has agreed or is obligated to pay for part of all of a recipient's health care services.

Thought content   Thought content generally refers to types of thoughts the client experiences. The MSE often includes questions regarding obsessions, compulsions, phobias, suicidality, homocidality, and antisocial thoughts.

Thought disorder   A thought disorder encompasses disorders of thought or perception such as Schizophrenia or Psychotic Disorders.

Thought disturbances   Thought disturbances are thoughts that are intrusive such as delusions (persecutory, grandeur, and somatic) or ideas of reference (thought broadcasting, thought control, or bizarre thoughts).

Thought processes   The manner in which thoughts are interconnected. It is measured in the MSE by aspects of the client's speech, such as number of ideas, flight of ideas, relevance, coherence, derailment, neologisms, and associations.

Treatment plan   A systematic plan, formulated by the client and therapist, in which the client's diagnosis, problem areas, goals and objectives, treatment strategies, and anticipated closure dates are delineated. It becomes an agreement, similar to a contract, for the course of therapy.

Utilization Review   An examination of the use and costs of medical service considering its appropriateness, efficiency, and level of treatment. It is typically referred to as an audit.

Bibliography

Allen, J. G., Buskirk, J. R., & Sebastian, L. M. (1992). A psychodynamic approach to the master treatment plan. *Bulletin of the Menninger Clinic, 56,* 487–510.

American Psychiatric Association. (2000). *Diagnostic and statistical manual of mental disorders* (4th ed., text revision). Washington, DC: American Psychiatric Association.

Barlow, D. H. (Ed.). (2001). *Clinical handbook of psychological disorders: A step-by-step treatment manual* (3rd ed.). New York: Guilford Press.

Brown, S. L. (1991). *The quality management professional's study guide.* Pasadena, CA: Managed Care Consultants.

Browning, C. H., & Browning, B. J. (1996). *How to partner with managed care.* New York: Wiley.

Commission on Accreditation of Rehabilitation Facilities. (2004). *Behavioral health standards manual.* Washington, DC: Commission on Accreditation of Rehabilitation Facilities.

Cohen, R. J. (1979). *Malpractice: A guide for mental health professionals.* New York: Free Press.

Dalton v. State. 308 N.Y.S. 2d 411 (1970).

Folstein, M. F., Folstein, S. E., & McHugh, P. R. (1975). Mini-mental state: A practical method for grading the cognitive state of patients for the clinician. *Journal of Psychiatric Research, 12,* 189–198.

Frederiksen, L. W., Richter, W. T., Jr., Johnoson, R. P., & Solomon, L. J. (1982). Specificity of performance feedback in a professional service delivery setting. *Journal of Organizational Behavior Management, 3,* 41–53.

Fulero, S. M., & Wilbert, J. R. (1998). Record keeping of clinical and counseling psychologists: A survey of practitioners. *Professional Psychology Research and Practice, 19,* 658–660.

Gabbard, G. O. (2000). *Psychodynamic psychiatry in clinical practice.* Washington, DC: American Psychiatric Press.

Galasso, D. (1987). Guidelines for developing multi-disciplinary treatment plans. *Hospitals and Community Psychiatry, 38,* 394–397.

Goldstein, G., & Hersen, M. (1990). *Handbook of psychological assessment* (2nd ed.). New York: Pergamon Press.

Goodman, M., Brown, J., & Dietz, P. (1996). *Managing managed care: A mental health practitioner's guide.* Washington, DC: American Psychiatric Press.

Grant, R. L. (1981). The capacity of the psychiatric record to meet changing needs. In C. Siegel & S. K. Fischer (Eds.), *Psychiatric records in mental health care.* New York: Brunner/Mazel.

Groth-Marnat, G. (2003). *Handbook of psychological assessment.* Hoboken, NJ: Wiley.

Gutheil, T. B., & Applebaum, P. S. (1982). *The clinical handbook of psychotherapy and the law.* New York: McGraw-Hill.

Hillard, J. R. (1995). Predicting Suicide. *Psychiatric Services, 46*(3), 223–225.

Howard, K. L., Orlinsky, D. E., & Lueger, R. J. (1994). The design of clinically relevant outcomes research: Some considerations and an example. In M. Aveline & D. Shapiro (Eds.), *Research foundations of psychotherapy services* (pp. 178–195). Sussex, England: Wiley.

Johnson v. United States. 409 F. Supp. 1283 (M.D. FA. 1976).

Joint Commission on Accreditation of Healthcare Organizations. (2004). *Standards for behavioral health care.* Oakbrook Terrace, IL: Joint Commission on Accreditation of Healthcare Organizations.

Jongsma, A. E., & Peterson, L. M. (2003). *The complete adult psychotherapy treatment planner* (3rd ed.). Hoboken, NJ: Wiley.

Jongsma, A. E., Peterson, L. M., & McInnis, W. P. (2000). *The adolescent psychotherapy treatment planner* (2nd ed.). New York: Wiley.

Jongsma, A. E., Peterson, L. M., & McInnis, W. P. (2003). *The child psychotherapy treatment planner* (3rd ed.). New York: Wiley.

Kennedy, J. A. (2003). *Fundamentals of psychiatric treatment planning.* Washington, DC: American Psychiatric Press.

Klopfer, W. G. (1960). *The psychological report.* New York: Grune & Stratton.

Lezak, M. D. (1995). *Neurological assessment* (3rd ed.). New York: Oxford University Press.

Lovett, S. B., Bosmajian, C. P., Frederiksen, L. W., & Elder, J. P. (1983). Monitoring professional service delivery: An organizational level intervention. *Behavior Therapy, 14,* 170–177.

Lyons, J. S., Howard, K. I., O'Mahoney, M. T., & Lish, J. D. (1997). *The measurement and management of clinical outcomes in mental health.* New York: Wiley.

Maltsberger, J. T. (1988). Suicide danger: Clinical estimation and decision. *Suicide and Life-Threatening Behavior, 18*(1), 47–54.

Maxmen, J. S., & Ward, N. G. (1995). *Essential psychopathology and its treatment.* New York: Norton.

Medicare program: Prospective payment for Medicare final rule. (1984). *Federal Register, 49,* 234–240.

Morrison, J. R. (1993). *The first interview.* New York: Guilford Press.

Morrison, J. R. (1995). DSM-IV *made easy.* New York: Guilford Press.

Ogles, B. M., Lambert, M. J., & Masters, K. S. (1996). *Assessing outcome in clinical practice.* Boston: Allyn & Bacon.

Orlinsky, D. E., & Howard, K. I. (1986). Process and outcome in psychotherapy. In S. L. Garfield & A. E. Bergin (Eds.), *Handbook of psychotherapy and behavior change* (3rd ed., pp. 217–234). New York: Wiley.

Ormiston, S., Barrett, N., Binder, R., & Molyneux, V. (1989). A partially computerized treatment plan. *Hospital and Community Psychology, 40,* 531–533.

Othmer, E., & Othmer, S. C. (2002). *The clinical interview using* DSM-IV-TR. Washington, DC: American Psychiatric Press.

Patterson, R., Cooke, C., & Liberman, R. (1972). Reinforcing the reinforcers: A method of supplying feedback to nursing personnel. *Behavior Therapy, 3,* 444–446.

Phares, E. J. (1988). *Clinical psychology: Concepts, methods, and profession* (3rd ed.). Pacific Grove, CA: Brooks/Cole.

Roth, A. D., & Fonagy, P. (2004). *What works for whom? A critical review of psychotherapy research* (2nd ed.). New York: Guilford Press.

Siegel, C., & Fischer, S. K. (1981). *Psychiatric records in mental health care.* New York: Bruner/Mazel.

Slovenko, R. (1979). On the need for record keeping in the practice of psychiatry. *Journal of Psychiatry and Law, 7,* 339–340.

Soisson, E. L., VandeCreek, L., & Knapp, S. (1987). Thorough record keeping: A good defense in a litigious era. *Professional Psychology: Research and Practice, 14,* 498–502.

Soreff, S. M., & McDuffee, M. A. (1993). *Documentation survival handbook: A clinician's guide to charting for better care, certification, reimbursement, and risk management.* Seattle, WA: Hogrefe & Huber.

Sperry, L., Brill, P., Howard, K. I., & Grisson, G. (1996). *Treatment outcomes in psychotherapy and psychiatric interventions.* New York: Brunner/Mazel.

Stout, C. E. (1997). *Psychological assessment in managed care*. New York: Wiley.

Sturm, I. E. (1987). The psychologist in the problem-oriented record (POR). *Professional Psychology Research and Practice, 18,* 155–158.

Trzepacz, P. T., & Baker, R. W. (1993). *The psychiatric MSE*. New York: Oxford University Press.

Walters, S. (1987). Computerized care plans help nurses achieve quality patient care. *Journal of Nursing Administration, 16,* 33–39.

Ware, J. E., Jr., & Hays, R. P. (1988). Methods for measuring patient satisfaction with specific medical encounters. *Medical Care, 26,* 393–402.

Wiger, D. E. (2005). *The clinical documentation sourcebook* (3rd ed.). New York: Wiley.

Wiger, D. E., and Harowski, K. J. (2003). *Essentials of crisis counseling and intervention*. New York: Wiley.

Wiger, D. E., and Huntley, D. K. (2002). *Essentials of interviewing*. New York: Wiley.

Wiger, D. E., and Solberg, K. B. (2001). *Tracking mental health outcomes*. New York: Wiley.

Wiley. (2003). *Thera*Scribe *4.0. The computerized assistant to the psychotherapy treatment planner*. New York: Wiley.

Zuckerman, E. L. (1997). *The paper office: Forms, guidelines, and resources* (2nd ed.). New York: Guilford Press.

Zuckerman, E. L. (2000). *Clinician's thesaurus: The guidebook for writing psychological reports* (5th ed.). New York: Guilford Press.

Index